Multimodal Psychiatric Music Therapy for Adults, Adolescents and Children

A Clinical Manual

Third Edition

Michael D. Cassity, Ph.D., MT-BC
and Julia E. Cassity, M.S., MT-BC, LPC, NCC

Jessica Kingsley Publishers
London and Philadelphia

Reprinted in 2006
by Jessica Kingsley Publishers
116 Pentonville Road
London N1 9JB, UK
and
400 Market Street, Suite 400
Philadelphia, PA 19106, USA

www.jkp.com

Copyright © Michael D. Cassity 2006

Previous edition published in 1991, 1994 by Michael Cassity, and in 1995 by MMB Music, Inc.
This edition first published by MMB Music, Inc. in 1998

Library of Congress Cataloging in Publication Data
A CIP catalog record for this book is available from the Library of Congress

British Library Cataloguing in Publication Data
A CIP catalogue record for this book is available from the British Library

ISBN-13: 978 1 84310 831 3
ISBN-10: 1 84310 831 3

Printed and bound in Great Britain by
Athenaeum Press, Gateshead, Tyne and Wear

CONTENTS

PART I

Chapter 1
ABOUT THIS MANUAL

Chapter 2
TUTORIAL GUIDE: Use of This Manual

PART II

Chapter 3
ADULTS

BEHAVIOR

Chapter 4
ADOLESCENTS

BEHAVIOR

AFFECT

SENSORY

IMAGERY

COGNITIVE

INTERPERSONAL-SOCIALIZATION (includes Leisure Skills)

DRUGS (includes D-1.0 Substance Use Or Abuse)

Chapter 5
CHILDREN

BEHAVIOR

AFFECT

SENSORY

IMAGERY

COGNITIVE

INTERPERSONAL-SOCIALIZATION

Chapter 6
ADULTS – MUSIC BEHAVIOR

LISTENING TO MUSIC

SINGING

Chapter 7
ADOLESCENTS – MUSIC BEHAVIOR

LISTENING TO MUSIC

PLAYING INSTRUMENTS

IMPROVISING MUSIC

SINGING

COMPOSING MUSIC

LOCOMOTOR MOVEMENT TO MUSIC

Chapter 8
CHILDREN – MUSIC BEHAVIOR

PART III

Chapter 9
PRACTICE EXERCISES

Chapter 10
GROUP THERAPY

Chapter 11
BRIEF THERAPY: Short-Term Music Therapy

Appendix I

Appendix II

Appendix III

Appendix IV

References

ACKNOWLEDGMENTS

The authors wish to express appreciation to the Oklahoma State Regents for Higher Education, Edward Daniel Dill, Ph.D., and Charles W. Chapman, Ph.D., for funding the initial research that made the writing of this book possible. Appreciation also is expressed to the late Erwin H. Schneider, Ph.D., for his early technical assistance in researching assessment techniques. Acknowledgments also are in order to Jenifer Nail for clerical assistance, the Southwestern Oklahoma State University music therapy students for their assistance in research and data processing, and to the music therapy clinical training directors who furnished the initial data that made possible the writing of this manual. This manual is dedicated to Professor Emeritus Charles Braswell for his 36 years of service to the music therapy profession at Loyola University, New Orleans.

PART I

ABOUT THIS MANUAL and TUTORIAL GUIDE

CHAPTER 1

ABOUT THIS MANUAL

Origin of Data

This manual contains patient problems and music behavior music therapists assess and treat most frequently in clinical training facilities. The information was collected from a national survey of all AMTA-approved psychiatric clinical training facilities. Clinical training directors (CTDs) submitted 801 music therapy interventions for assessing and treating 200 patient problems, and 354 interventions for assessing music behavior. This manual reports the patient problems, music behaviors, and music therapy interventions according to the frequency with which they were reportedly used in clinical training facilities. For a summary and statistical analysis of information contained in this manual the reader is referred to the *Journal of Music Therapy* (Cassity & Cassity, 1994).

In brief, clinical training directors were given areas of nonmusic behavior that had been extracted from the music therapy literature and asked to choose the areas they assess and treat most frequently during music therapy sessions. Next they were asked to write, for each area they selected, two patient problems they assess and treat most frequently. Finally, for each of the patient problems they listed, they were requested to list two music therapy interventions they use most frequently to assess or treat the patient problems. A similar procedure was used to collect information about the assessment of music behavior and activity therapy assessment.

The patient problems and music therapy interventions in this manual are indexed by chronological age (CA) and level of functioning. Sex is an additional index with Adults. The CA levels are Adulthood, Adolescence, and Childhood. Infancy was not included because an insufficient number of CTDs worked with infants. Level of functioning indices were obtained by asking CTDs to rate their patients using the *Global Assessment of Functioning (GAF) Scale* as found in the *Diagnostic and Statistical Manual of Mental Disorders III-R (DSM-III-R)* (APA, 1987). The GAF Scale was later republished in the *DSM-IV* (APA, 1994).

The GAF Scale as originally published in the DSM-III-R ranged from *1*, representing the most severe symptoms, to *90*, representing the mildest symptoms (the GAF Scale in the DSM-IV is extended upward to *100*). The GAF Scale was arranged into nine ten-point intervals, with nine of the intervals containing a verbal descriptor of typical patient symptoms (in the DSM-IV, a tenth interval, *91–100*, was added to describe healthy behavior and no symptoms). CTDs were asked to indicate, using the GAF Scale, the level of functioning typical of the majority of patients treated in their clinical training programs. The numbers following each music therapy intervention in this manual are GAF Scale scores. Each number, or score, indicates the level of functioning of the patients with whom the CTD used the intervention. For interventions having more than one GAF Scale score, the number of GAF Scale scores listed equals the number of times the intervention was submitted by different CTDs. For example, 30-40-35 indicates the intervention was submitted by three CTDs, and that the intervention was used with patients having GAF Scale scores of 30, 40, and 35. With adult patients, the GAF Scale scores are preceded by the letter *M* (Male) or *F* (Female), indicating the sex of the patient for whom the intervention was designed.

Data also were collected on the mean GAF of patients for whom this manual was designed. The mean GAF rating of adult patients was 36.5 with a median of 33. Seventy percent of the CTDs indicated the GAF level of their adult patients to be between 21 and 40. The following description applies to patients with a GAF rating of 31–40, therefore approximating the typical adult treated in psychiatric music therapy clinical training programs:

> Some impairment in reality testing or communication (e.g., speech is at times illogical, obscure, or irrelevant) or major impairment in several areas, such as work or school, family relations, judgment, thinking, or mood (e.g., depressed man avoids friends, neglects family, and is unable to work; child frequently beats up younger children, is defiant at home, and is failing at school) (APA, 1994, p. 32).

CTDs gave somewhat higher GAF ratings to their adolescent than to their adult patients. When asked to indicate, using the GAF, the level of functioning typical of the majority of adolescents treated in their clinical training program, 87% of the CTDs indicated the level of their adolescents to be between 31 and 50. The mean GAF rating was 40.5 and the median was 41. The level of functioning of the typical adolescent treated in psychiatric music therapy clinical training programs therefore would border between the above descriptor and the following for patients with a GAF of 41 to 50:

> Serious symptoms (e.g., suicidal ideation, severe obsessional rituals, frequent shoplifting) OR any serious impairment in social, occupational, or school functioning (e.g., no friends, unable to keep a job) (APA, 1994, p. 32).

Children were given the highest GAF ratings. Although 71% of all children were given GAF ratings of between 33 and 50, the mean GAF was 45.76 and the median was 45. The above descriptor therefore would approximate patients treated in psychiatric music therapy clinical training programs who were in the CA level of childhood.

Evolution of the Model

During the questionnaire analysis difficulties emerged relating to certain assessment areas and music conditions CTDs had chosen. Table A on the following page illustrates the original areas CTDs chose for adult male and female patients, and the number and percentage of CTDs choosing the areas.

Certain assessment areas in Table A, which had been extracted from the music therapy literature, and which had been chosen most frequently by music therapists, were lacking in specificity. These assessment areas therefore, did not adequately define the type of problem they were to assess. An example was the assessment area, Coping. Although approximately 55% (female and male combined data) of the CTDs indicated they assessed Coping, the specific problems for Coping could have been classified within a variety of assessment areas. Thirty-two percent of the problems listed under Coping were Affective problems, 21% were Interpersonal-Socialization problems, and 29% were Cognitive problems. The highest inter-therapist agreement as to the meaning of Coping therefore, was 32%. Coping as an assessment area was too general and did not adequately refer to a specific area of assessment.

TABLE A

AREAS ASSESSED MOST FREQUENTLY IN PSYCHIATRIC CLINICAL TRAINING FACILITIES

ASSESSMENT AREA (ADULT FEMALE PATIENTS, N = 41)	n	%
Affect	31	75.61
Socialization	26	63.42
Coping Skills	22	53.66
Interpersonal	19	46.34
Leisure Skills	15	36.59
Communication	13	31.71
Behavior	12	29.27
Substance Use or Abuse	11	26.83
Cognitive	7	17.07
Psychological	7	17.07

ASSESSMENT AREA (ADULT MALE PATIENTS, N = 35)	n	%
Affect	26	74.29
Socialization	22	62.86
Leisure Skills	20	57.14
Coping	20	57.14
Interpersonal	18	51.43
Communication	15	42.86
Behavior	10	28.57
Cognitive	8	22.86
Psychological	7	20.00
Mental Functioning	5	14.29
Substance Use or Abuse	5	14.29
Sensory Integrative Functioning	3	8.57
Imagery	2	5.71
Physical Well-Being	2	5.71

(Inter-therapist agreement was used in this study as an index for quantifying the degree of meaningfulness to CTDs of a given assessment area. Inter-therapist agreement used in this sense refers to the percentage of CTDs who described the same type of problem for a given assessment area. Examples are illustrated above, and in the following text).

Similar "catch-all" assessment areas that had to be discarded were Mental Functioning and Psychological with respective inter-therapist agreements of 53% and 50%. The assessment area of Communication was another example of an assessment category with low inter-therapist agreement. When CTDs wrote specific problems for Communication, 48% were Interpersonal-Socialization problems (e.g., does not verbally interact with others), and 25% were Affective problems such as the inability to identify or express emotion. Other problems and music conditions written for Communication were physical speech problems. Communication, therefore, was restricted to physical speech problems since the areas of Interpersonal-Socialization (85% inter-therapist agreement) and Affect (84% inter-therapist agreement) already existed for classifying interpersonal and affective problems. The problems and music conditions which had been written for the nonspecific areas discussed above therefore were reclassified into already existing assessment areas having the highest inter-therapist agreement and to which they were related. Affective problems, for example, were classified under Affect.

Because of the similarity of the types of problems written for the areas of Interpersonal and Socialization, these areas were combined. Because of the close relationship of Leisure Skills to Interpersonal-Socialization, and because of the 85% inter-therapist agreement as to the meaning of Leisure Skills, Leisure Skills was classified as a separate area within Interpersonal-Socialization.

Selecting a Model. Because of the above inadequacies of existing assessment areas extracted from the music therapy literature, the need emerged for a systematic therapeutic model for classifying the patient problems and interventions submitted by CTDs. A model into which all patient problems could be classified was the Multimodal Therapy model (Lazarus, 1976; 1989). In addition, the Multimodal model previously had been recommended for use in music therapy (Adleman, 1985), and used as a model for music therapy practice (Cassity & Theobold, 1990).

The Multimodal model involves comprehensive assessment and intervention across a person's BASIC I.D. (or basic identity). We, at base, are biochemical and neurophysiological beings. "Our personalities are the products of our ongoing *Behaviors, Affective Processes, Sensations, Images, Cognitions, Interpersonal Relationships,* and *Biological Functions*" (Lazarus, p. 13). All these factors forming the BASIC I.D., must be considered when assessing the total person. To form a sensible acronym, Lazarus labeled the biological modality "D" for drugs. BASIC ID, therefore, stands for the basic identity of a person. According to Lazarus,

> The BASIC I.D. represents the fundamental vectors of human personality just as ABCDEFG represents the notes in music. There are no HIJKLMNOP. Combinations of ABCDEFG (with some sharps or flats) will yield everything from "chopsticks" to Mozart (Lazarus, 1989, p. 16).

Thus, Lazarus hypothesized that the BASIC I.D. model can account for every condition a person encounters.

Description of the Model

Following are descriptions of each multimodal category with examples of clinical issues that may appropriately be addressed within each category.

The category of *Behavior* refers mainly to overt behaviors such as acts, habits, gestures, and reactions that are measurable and observable. The therapist may be concerned with behaviors that are interfering with the patient's happiness, what the patient would like to start doing, or what he or she would like to do more of, or do less of. In adult psychiatric music therapy, lack of assertiveness, lack of attention span, and poor eye contact are examples of behaviors of frequent concern to music therapists.

Affect refers to emotions, moods, or strong feelings. The therapist may be concerned with emotions the patient experiences most often, unwanted emotions, or no emotion. Affective problems are the most frequent type of problem CTDs assess with adolescents, and the second most frequent problem assessed with adults. With adolescents, for example, CTDs are most concerned with emotions such as the inability to identify or express feelings, inappropriate expression of feelings, anger or rage, stress reactions, and excessive anxiety.

Sensation refers to the five senses: seeing, hearing, touching, tasting, and smelling. The therapist may note negative sensations experienced by the patient such as tension, pain, dizziness, sweating, blushing, and "butterflies" in stomach. What the patient likes to taste, smell, hear, or see also may be of concern. Although CTDs assess and treat sensory disorders relatively infrequently, when they do treat them, the treatment usually involves the use of relaxation techniques with patients who are having problems coping with stress and tension.

Imagery may include recurring dreams; vivid memories that may be bothersome or troubling, the patient's self image or body image (how does the patient describe his or her self-image, "pictures" of the past, present, and future that may be troubling, and "auditory images" such as tunes or sounds heard repeatedly that are a problem). Although imagery is another infrequent assessment area in music therapy, when it is assessed it is usually during guided imagery or relaxation. The music therapist may be concerned with whether the patient can envision and focus on a pleasant place during guided imagery or relaxation. With battered women, imagery is assessed because of its importance at promoting ventilation, relaxation, and the alleviation of anxiety during relaxation and guided imagery sessions (Cassity & Theobold, 1990).

Cognitive refers to ideas, values, opinions, and attitudes that interfere with the patient's happiness. The therapist may be concerned with the patient's negative self-statements, irrational ideas (What are the patient's shoulds, oughts, and musts?), and the patient's cherished beliefs and values. Cognitive problems are the third most frequent type of problem CTDs assess with adults and adolescents, and a second most frequent problem assessed with children. With adult patients, music therapists most frequently are concerned with cognitive problems such as low self-esteem as evidenced by negative self statements, deficit problem solving skills, lack of reality orientation, poor short- or long-term memory skills, and poor decision-making skills.

Interpersonal includes problems the patient has with other people and concerns they have about the way they are treated by others. In psychiatric music therapy, Interpersonal-Socialization is the most frequent area assessed with adults and children, and the second most frequent area of assessment with adolescents. With adult patients CTDs most frequently are concerned with reclusive, withdrawn, or isolative behavior, inappropriate use of leisure time, uncooperative behavior, a lack of interest in or lack of motivation to use leisure time, and difficulty bonding with others.

Drugs refers to any concerns the patient has about his or her state of health, or the physical well-being of the patient. Such concerns could relate to the patient's habits pertaining to diet, exercise, and fitness. In addition, Drugs could refer to medications or drugs taken by the patient, substance abuse, and to drug side effects. In psychiatric music therapy, Drugs is the fourth most frequent area of assessment with adults and adolescents, and the second most frequent area of assessment with children. The assessment of Drugs with children most frequently focuses on physical well-being, such as gross and fine motor coordination, and physical communication problems, such as impaired ability to describe objects, feelings, or situations.

Multimodal therapy is very eclectic. It does not adhere to just one mode of therapy such as Gestalt therapy or Behavior therapy, but rather, it includes a whole gamut of therapies. The inherent eclecticism of the model makes it especially amenable for use in music therapy because of the wide diversity in music therapy practice (all chronological ages and diagnoses), and because music therapists work in settings representative of many different schools of psychotherapy. Interventions a music therapist might implement, such as relaxation training, aerobic exercises, rational-emotive therapy, and assertiveness training all could be used as treatments in a multimodal profile.

It is very important to remember that although multimodal assessment and treatment attends to specific problems, each within a given modality, it also focuses on the interaction between a given modality and the other modalities. Thus, a problem in one modality will influence problems in all other areas or modalities. This can be illustrated by the following example:

- Laura has trouble asserting herself (Behavior).
- She feels frustrated (Affect).
- She experiences life as being extremely stressful resulting in feelings of chronic fatigue (Sensation).
- She fantasizes how she could "get even" (Imagery).
- She believes others are always taking advantage of her by manipulating her into doing what they would like to do instead of doing what she would like to do. (Cognitive).
- She sometimes acts in a passive-aggressive manner with her friends (Interpersonal).
- She abuses alcohol and prescription medication to decrease feelings of fatigue (Drugs).

Laura's not being assertive results in a whole array of problems under the BASIC I.D. We can tell a lot about what is going on in Laura's life by looking at each area.

When assessing each modality it is essential to go back and determine the effect of one area upon all the others. For example, after assessing the affect it is important to determine what the patient tends to do or how he/she behaves when feeling a certain way. For example, to a patient who is experiencing a lot of anxiety, the music therapist should say, "How do you behave when you are very anxious?" "What happens?"

Likewise, when assessing Sensory, after determining applicable sensations you go backwards and note how the sensations caused the patient to act or feel, and so on. For example, when sensations occur such as hyperventilation or muscle tension, ask the patient "How does that make you feel?" "What does that make you do?" So, as you go down the BASIC I.D. you may have to go back up the BASIC I.D.

Therefore, all modalities are very interdependent. By understanding the interactions among them, one is better able to achieve a thorough and holistic understanding of the person.

Functional analysis. In addition to examining the interactions among the modalities, the therapist should investigate the antecedent stimuli in a given situation, organismic or mediating variables, the subject's observable response, and the consequences. This procedure involves asking the patient *What, When, Where, Who,* and *How* questions such as the above. *Why* questions are not as productive in terms of yielding clinically relevant information (Bandler & Grinder; 1975). Asking *Why* questions frequently produces patient rationalization. According to Egan, the cause, especially remote causes, are seldom evident. Asking the patient to explain "...causes often is inviting them to whistle in the wind" (Egan, 1990, p. 161).

Modality firing order. Lazarus refers to modality firing order as the sequence with which the BASIC I.D. modalities are exhibited during a given response pattern. Examining the interactive pattern of the modalities for purposes of determining the sequence of the firing order is referred to as *tracking.* For example, as indicated above, Laura's modality firing order was Behavior, Affect, Sensory, Imagery, Cognitive, Interpersonal, and finally, drugs. The Behavior (lack of assertiveness) produced the Affect, the Affect resulted in the Sensory, and etc. Not all modality firing orders, however, follow the BASIC I.D. sequence. Ron, for example had very low self-esteem. He frequently made negative self-statements and lacked the self-confidence to try to overcome life problems or to try new activities (Cognitive). He projected his low self-opinion onto others by frequently saying undesirable things about other patients and staff, resulting in peer rejection (Interpersonal). During conversation with others he had poor eye contact (Behavior). He fantasized himself as "one of the little people" and being "walked on" by others who always "come out on top" (Imagery). Following the imagery Ron recalled several sad experiences, and expressed hopelessness and pessimism about the future (Affect). Ron's modality firing order was Cognitive, Interpersonal, Behavior, Imagery, and Affect.

Affective responses or emotional disturbances therefore, can be triggered by a sequence of events. The sequence may begin with any modality (e.g., a person can dwell on thoughts and images that lead to unpleasant sensations, which may in turn lead to behavior). There is a close interaction among the various modalities. The way we feel, think, behave, etc., affects our biochemical and neurophysiological makeup, or what's going on in our body. The "Drug" modality in turn, can affect the other modalities. It is therefore important to examine the firing order, or the sequence that the modalities are exhibited during a response pattern.

Uni or bimodal interventions. At times a patient's BASIC I.D. may not reveal a network of interrelated problems, or the patient may respond poorly to multifaceted intervention and insists on working on one or two problems. Although a multimodal assessment usually is recommended, the therapist and patient may choose to work on one or two clear-cut problems in such situations. If therapeutic progress is not made however, or if the patient is given an ambiguous or faltering diagnosis, a multimodal assessment may prove helpful.

Structural profiles. Structural profiles sometimes are constructed during the initial assessment phase. Some people may tend to be feelers, thinkers, doers, fantasizers, etc. The patient who is primarily a thinker, for example, may prefer to work on cognitive problems rather than in other modalities. Such knowledge may assist the therapist in structuring the therapeutic session to elicit greater involvement from the patient. The process of treating problems within a patient's preferred modality before delving into more clinically relevant problems within less preferred modalities is referred to as *bridging.*

Lazarus (1989) uses the *Structural Profile Inventory* to determine the structural profile of patients. The *Structural Profile Inventory* provides information on the extent to which patients operate in the various modalities. The Profile consists of 35 statements, each related to a given modality within the BASIC I.D. The patient rates each item on a scale of 1 (Strongly Disagree) to 7 (Strongly Agree). Profile results can then be analyzed graphically, usually using a histogram, to indicate the extent that the patient is functioning in each modality.

The patient, therapist, or both may draw up a structural profile. If the patient is assigned to do their own structural profile it is recommended they be provided with a written description of each modality area in the BASIC I.D. as given above.

Group therapy. According to Lazarus, multimodal therapy may be conducted as group therapy. Lonely, isolated individuals who need the opportunity to make friends benefit considerably from group therapy. Multimodal group therapy may be especially appropriate for music therapy since a major music therapy goal is the development of interpersonal relationships. Poor candidates for group therapy are patients who are severely depressed, paranoid, delusional, or who have ritualistic obsessive compulsive characteristics.

Lazarus recommends certain procedures and principles of group therapy. During the first session, patients are helped to feel more at ease if a discussion is conducted about the benefits of group therapy. During the second session patients are helped to construct their own modality profiles. The remainder of the sessions are devoted to working on each patient's problems as specified in her modality profile. After the group members become experienced with multimodal therapy, they usually derive benefit from tracking their modality firing order. Finally, Lazarus recommends that group therapy sessions be time limited. If groups are told that therapy will be concluded for example, after 25 sessions, the group usually achieves more.

Second-order BASIC I.D.[5] A Second-order BASIC I.D. is sometimes constructed when therapeutic progress falters because of a persistent patient problem within a given modality. For example in the above case of Laura, therapeutic goals may be to increase assertiveness, decrease feelings of frustration, and so on, down her BASIC I.D. If however, therapeutic progress falters because of her increasing alcohol abuse, a second-order BASIC I.D. may need to be constructed to focus exclusively on her alcohol abuse:

B. Drinks excessively at local bar and at home.
A. Experiences depression as a result of drinking.
S. Has migraine headaches as a result of alcohol abuse.
I. Imagines she is in total control of her drinking; fantasizes her bar life as glamorous.
C. Denies having a drinking problem.
I. Increasing interpersonal problems are the fault of others (e.g., inconsiderate boss); associates with bar crowd.
D. Alcohol abuse has dramatically increased.

Finally, it should be emphasized that Lazarus has documented impressive outcomes and follow-ups using the multimodal approach to assessment and treatment. Possibly by using this systematic approach in the field of psychiatric music therapy we can experience more success in the assessment and treatment of our patients.

Most Frequent Modalities in Psychiatric Music Therapy
During the initial assessment phase it may be most productive to assess first the modalities assessed most frequently by CTDs. CTDs prefer to assess and treat certain modalities significantly more frequently than others with adults ($X^2 = 298.20$; $p < .001$), adolescents ($X^2 = 126.27$; $p < .001$), and children ($X^2 = 39.79$; $p < .001$). As indicated in Tables B, C, and D, 76% of all adult problems and 85% of all adolescent problems assessed or treated by CTDs were either Interpersonal, Affective, or Cognitive problems. With children, Interpersonal, Behavior, Cognitive, and Physical (including motor and receptive and expressive language) problems accounted for 82% of all problems assessed or treated by CTDs.

TABLE B

MODALITIES ASSESSED AND TREATED MOST FREQUENTLY IN PSYCHIATRIC MUSIC THERAPY CLINICAL TRAINING FACILITIES: ADULTS

MODALITY	NUMBER OF PROBLEMS ASSESSED	% OF PROBLEMS
Interpersonal	177	33.27
Affect	121	22.37
Cognitive	112	20.70
Behavior	55	10.17
Drugs	54	9.98
Sensory	20	3.70
Imagery	2	00.37
	541	100.56

TABLE C

MODALITIES ASSESSED AND TREATED MOST FREQUENTLY IN PSYCHIATRIC MUSIC THERAPY CLINICAL TRAINING FACILITIES: ADOLESCENTS

MODALITY	NUMBER OF PROBLEMS ASSESSED	% OF PROBLEMS
Affect	51	32.69
Interpersonal	49	31.41
Cognitive	32	20.51
Drugs	12	7.69
Behavior	11	7.05
Imagery	1	00.64
Sensory	0	00.00
	156	99.99

TABLE D

MODALITIES ASSESSED AND TREATED MOST FREQUENTLY IN PSYCHIATRIC MUSIC THERAPY CLINICAL TRAINING FACILITIES: CHILDREN

MODALITY	NUMBER OF PROBLEMS ASSESSED	% OF PROBLEMS
Interpersonal	32	30.77
Behavior	18	17.31
Drugs	18	17.31
Cognitive	18	17.31
Affect	10	9.62
Sensory	6	5.77
Imagery	2	1.92
	104	100.01

CHAPTER 2

TUTORIAL GUIDE
Use of This Manual

Initial Assessment

During the initial assessment phase, in addition to using music to establish rapport, the patient's life history is reviewed, the patient is interviewed to determine present problems, and the *Psychiatric Music Therapy Questionnaire (PMTQ)* is administered. This information is then used to construct the patient's multimodal profile.

Information concerning life history may be determined by reviewing assessments given by other professionals such as the social worker or psychologist. Music therapists who do not have access to assessments given by other professionals may obtain life history information by administering the *Multimodal Life History Questionnaire* (Lazarus, 1989).

After interviewing the patients about their present life situations, the PMTQ is administered. There are three PMTQs, one each for adults (Appendix I), adolescents (Appendix II), and children (Appendix III). The PMTQs for adults and adolescents are administered by interviewing the patient, and the PMTQ for children is administered by interviewing a significant second person, such as the child's parent.

The PMTQs are designed to provide intake information concerning problems most frequently treated using music therapy. Items in each PMTQ are indexed to specific problems addressed in this treatment manual. An example of the indexing is illustrated in the PMTQ for adolescents on page 224 of Appendix II. The "(A-1)" after the first item, "Other people know when I am happy, sad, or excited (A-1)" indicates the item, and any other item following it, is a measure of the "Inability to identify/express feelings...," the first problem (A-1) listed under adolescent Affect on page vi of the Table of Contents. The Table of Contents in turn, refers the reader to page 86 under adolescent Affect in the manual, where music therapy interventions are listed for treating the "Inability to identify/express feelings...." If the music therapist decides to use one of the interventions, the intervention is written in the patient's multimodal music therapy profile.

The PMTQ requires patients to rate themselves on a five-point scale, with "1" indicating "Strongly Disagree" and "5" indicating they "Strongly Agree." Generally, PMTQ items rated "4" or "5" are considered to be indicative of patient problems, and therefore should be included in the multimodal music therapy profile. An exception is with items having a reversed scale that are stated in the positive rather than in the negative. For these items a patient rating of "1" or "2" would generally be the criterion for inclusion in the multimodal music therapy profile.

The assessment areas in the PMTQs are not presented in the same order as in the BASIC I.D. or the manual, but rather according to the frequency that they are assessed and treated by music therapists. For example, Chapter 1 indicated that with adolescents, music therapists most frequently assess and treat affective problems, followed by interpersonal, cognitive, etc. This order therefore, was the one used for the assessment areas in the PMTQ for adolescents.

Following is a summary of the initial assessment procedure: (1) Review the patient's case history; (2) Administer the PMTQ that is appropriate for the patient's chronological age level; (3) Construct a BASIC I.D. to get the *big picture* of the patient's problems and to compare the agreement of PMTQ results with case history results; (4) Construct a multimodal music therapy profile from the PMTQ results. Because of the unique needs of different patients, this manual should not be used as a cookbook approach to music therapy. The music therapist therefore may choose *not* to select interventions from this manual for inclusion in the multimodal music therapy profile.

Program Planning

Once the initial assessment has been conducted, goals, objectives, and implementation strategies may be planned. The implementation strategy provides information concerning the materials needed, type of reinforcement, therapist behavior, and patient behavior. Progress is then charted and evaluated in the session/monthly progress report.

Case Example: Adults

The following case of *D* provides an example of how to derive a multimodal analysis from the initial assessment.

Case of *D*

DATE: October 13, 1995

D is a 35-year-old male receiving support services at a community mental health center. According to *D*, his mother had schizophrenia, and his grandmother took responsibility for him. At age three *D* was placed in a Masonic home. During childhood *D* was sexually and physically abused from age three on, and had no church affiliation. *D* later stated that during this time he "learned to show no feelings." By age 16 *D* was drinking heavily, taking illegal street drugs, and recalled that he "had no family." At age 19 he was placed in a metropolitan crisis center. *D* never married and was rejected by the military.

Despite these difficulties *D* did garner some achievements. He graduated from high school, then attended the University of Oklahoma for three years as a Russian studies major. In Russian studies he was described as being a bright student with grades averaging a B⁺. During his senior year he transferred to a regional university as a psychology major. Although the WAIS-R indicated he had an IQ of 80, the quotient probably was inaccurate because of his psychosis. *D* was beginning to experience symptoms of schizophrenia. At age 22, *D* was employed as an aide at a state psychiatric hospital where he remained for 10 years. *D* reported spending his leisure time engaging in reading or "doing nothing."

When *D* was 34, he was admitted to a state hospital (different from the one where he had been employed) for treatment of schizophrenia. Several months later he was referred to a community mental health center with the goal of community placement. It was recommended that *D* first be placed in a transitional lodge, then given continuous community support services to prevent further hospital returns and episodes of active schizophrenia. At the community mental health center he was described as having poor leisure skills (no hobbies), lacking in daily living skills, having poor personal hygiene, withdrawn, severely depressed, and passive. Other assessments revealed that although *D* had been a bright student, his speech (thought processes) was characterized by slowness, blocking, hesitancy, incoherence, simplicity, and concreteness. His thought content was suicidal, evidenced guilt, disturbed by recurring fantasies (which he would not discuss), and high in persecutory beliefs and hallucinatory perceptions. Immediate retention and recall were adequate, but short term and long term memory was inadequate. *D* was given the following diagnosis:

Axis I: 295.70   Schizoaffective Disorder.
          305.00   Alcohol Abuse.
Axis II: 301.9   Personality Disorder NOS (Not Otherwise Specified)
Axis III: None
Axis IV: Psychosocial and Environmental Problems: Repeated physical sexual abuse.
Axis V: Current GAF: 50; flat affect; moderate difficulty in social functioning.

After reviewing *D's* history and administering the PMTQ for adults, the following BASIC I.D. was compiled from the case history and PMTQ results to provide a systematic and comprehensive overview of *D's* problems.

BASIC I.D.

MODALITY	PROBLEMS
Behavior	Lack of assertiveness; has difficulty expressing own views on a topic during group discussion; passive.
Affect	Feelings of anger and stress. Depressed
Sensation	Hallucinatory perceptions
Imagery	Recurring fantasies that *D* will not discuss
Cognitive	Low self-esteem, low self-opinion, lack of self-confidence Poor short- and long-term memory Persecutory beliefs Suicidal thought content
Interpersonal	Reclusive, withdrawn, isolative Poor leisure skills Difficulty maintaining long term relationships
Drugs	Haldol: 10 mg. each evening, 150 mg. once a month Cogentin: 2 mg. per day Benedryl: 50 mg at night Absence of daily exercise, poor muscle tone. Substance abuse history Poor personal hygiene

Following construction of the above BASIC I.D., *D's* Multimodal Music Therapy Profile was constructed. The purpose of the multimodal profile is to target problems for music therapy intervention, and to specify the type of music therapy intervention to be used. The problems in the profile are the types of problems music therapists most commonly treat, as indicated in this manual, as well as individualized problems for which *D* is in need of treatment.

Multimodal Music Therapy Profile: *D*

I. MUSIC PREFERENCES

D's favorite type of music is Jazz. When he was asked who his favorite jazz performer was he said "B. B. King." He also likes popular rock of the 1950s and 1960s, religious, and classical. Neutral responses were given in the areas of popular and country music. He dislikes folk music. He did not indicate a preference for a favorite performer or composer. *D* would very much like to learn to play the saxophone or guitar, and likes to participate in group sing-a-longs accompanied by a pianist or guitarist.

II. MULTIMODAL PROBLEM ANALYSIS

Interpersonal	Problem	Music Therapy Intervention
IS-1	**Reclusive, withdrawn, isolative**	• Elicit patient discussion of song characteristics during music listening. • Play socialization games such as "Stop the Music." • Instrumental or improvisation group requiring nonverbal and verbal interaction with others (e.g., leading the group, listening to and responding to others).
IS-2	Poor leisure skills	• Determine specific style(s) of jazz preferred as well as other music preferences. • Provide leisure education (e.g., community music and nonmusic activities, building a tape library). • Take on field trips to community music events.
IS-5	**Difficulty maintaining long term relationships**	• Encourage patient bonding during above group singing and instrumental groups. • During above listening-discussion group, use songs that focus on positive aspects of relationships and friendships.

Affect	Problem	Music Therapy Intervention
A-3	**Feelings of anger and stress**	• During above listening-discussion group, from a list of titles expressing frustration, have patient select a title that expresses his feelings. Use techniques in manual to encourage expression of source of anger.

Cognitive	Problem	Music Therapy Intervention
C-1	**Low self-esteem, low self-opinion, lack of self-confidence**	• Engineer the above instrumental music therapy activities to produce patient feelings of success, accomplishment, and peer acceptance. • Use success oriented music activities or lessons. Ask patient to point out positive aspects of their playing.

C-5	Poor short- and long-term memory involving time, place, names and events	• During the above group singing activity, ask the patient to identify his favorite song, the name of the song just sung, questions about song lyrics, musical characteristics (e.g., tempo, melody), etc. • Promote recognition of names of peers.

Behavior	Problem	Music Therapy Intervention
B-1	Lack of assertiveness, has difficulty expressing own views on a topic during group discussion.	• During above listening-discussion activity, have the patient identify assertive and non-assertive messages in the song lyrics. • Engineer group situations in which the patient must negotiate with another patient (e.g., which song to play or sing). • Have patients list things they enjoy most. Then communicate them to the group (Song: "My Favorite Things").

Drugs	Problem	Music Therapy Intervention
D-1.2	Check for possible denial of substance	• Use song discussion techniques for detecting denial (see manual, abuse problem, page 79).
D-2.1	Absence of daily exercise, poor muscle tone	• Involve the patient in regular rhythmic exercise.
Medication	Haldol: 10 mg. each evening, 150 mg. once a month, Cogentin: 2 mg. per day, Benedryl: 50 mg. at night	• Observe for possible medication side effects.

III. POST INTERVIEW OBSERVATIONS

D had good concentration, attention span, and retention. He appeared to be physically out of shape, had a flat affect, and projected low self-confidence and self-concept. He seemed to have a favorable attitude toward participation in music therapy.

In the above multimodal analysis, the column on the left indicates the modality or area of assessment, the center column refers to the patient's problem, and the right column is the music therapy intervention used to treat the problem. Letter numbers in the left column under each area of assessment refer to the order that problems are listed under each modality in the manual, and in the Table of Contents. For example, the letter number IS-1 is written under "Interpersonal," and to the left of "Reclusive, Withdrawn, Isolative" in the above modality analysis. Page v of the Table of Contents indicates reclusive, withdrawn, isolative is the first, or most frequent problem music therapists treat in the Interpersonal-Socialization modality, and that the problem can be found on page 67. On page 67 "Reclusive, Withdrawn, Isolative behavior" is listed and is followed by the types of music therapy interventions used most frequently to treat the problem. Likewise, the letter number A-3 under Affect in the above modality analysis refers to the third problem listed under Affect on page iv of the Table of Contents, "Becomes angry when coping with frustration." This problem is listed on page 53 and is followed by the music therapy interventions used most frequently to treat the problem.

Also in the above multimodal analysis, the problems in bold lettering were problems that D indicated were most severe. A perusal of the above multimodal analysis indicates a predominance of such problems. Because of the preponderance of problems which D rated as a "4" or "5" in the PMTQ, it was decided to focus on D's most severe problems. To list all the problems would have made the profile unmanageable resulting in an overly ambitious music therapy treatment plan. Also, an examination of the PMTQ results revealed that in most cases, the lesser problems were probably being exacerbated by the more severe problems. Eagan (1990) uses the term *leverage* to refer to the process of ameliorating lesser problems by targeting more severe or primary patient problems. One problem listed which was rated a "4" was "poor leisure skills." Leisure skills were targeted because of the possibility that they might directly enhance chances for improvement in the other areas targeted, by contributing to D's life satisfaction, self-confidence, and socialization.

Another problem, "Substance Use," was included in D's profile even though it was rated a "3." D gave a neutral response to the PMTQ item, "I do not have a substance abuse problem." This may indicate D either believes he has been rehabilitated, or that he cannot admit he has a substance abuse problem (denial). Also, this statement apparently is the only PMTQ response that is inconsistent with D's case history and diagnosis. It was therefore decided to use music therapy to attempt to determine whether D was denying having a substance abuse problem.

Because D had many problems that are treated frequently in music therapy, and because of D's music preferences, D was accepted for music therapy. The following intervention plan and implementation strategy are representative of the first ones constructed for D. They focus on the first music therapy intervention listed in D's Multimodal Profile (above) for his reclusive and withdrawn behavior.

MUSIC THERAPY INTERVENTION PLAN

NAME: _D_   CASE NO: _0001_
DATE OF ASSESSMENT: _10-30-95_

Music Therapy Goals and Objectives

Goal #1: Interpersonal-Isolation
Goal Statement: _D will demonstrate socialization skills by 2-1-96._

Objective #1.1 Objective Statement: _During music listening, D will verbalize more than a yes or no response in discussion, when prompted by the therapist, in 4 out of 5 sessions by 11-30-95._

Person Responsible: _John Doe, MT-BC_
Date Started: _11-02-95_   Date Ended: _____
Reason Ended: _____

Objective #1.2 Objective Statement: <u>During music listening, *D* will spontaneously verbalize more</u> <u>than a yes or no response in discussion of selected music, in 4 out of 5 sessions by 1-05-96.</u>

Person Responsible: *John Doe, MT-BC*
Date Started: <u>12-06-95</u>   Date Ended: _____
Reason Ended: _____

Objective #1.3 Objective Statement: <u>[NOTE: Record any future socialization objectives for</u> <u>Goal #1 here.]</u>

Person Responsible: _____
Date Started: _____   Date Ended: _____
Reason Ended: _____

Following construction of the intervention plan, implementation strategies are constructed. Following is an example of an implementation strategy.

IMPLEMENTATION STRATEGY

NAME: *D*_____   CASE NO: <u>0001</u>
DATE OF ASSESSMENT: <u>10-30-95</u>_____

Objective #1.1: <u>During music listening, *D* will verbalize more than a yes or no response in</u> <u>discussion, when prompted by the therapist, in 4 out of 5 sessions by 11-30-95.</u>

Materials Needed: <u>Guitar or piano, B. B. King recordings, '50s and '60s rock music selected by *D*.</u>

Reinforcement Schedule: <u>Continuous verbal reinforcement in sessions 1–10.</u>

THERAPIST BEHAVIOR	PATIENT BEHAVIOR
• Ask *D* to select a song he would like to hear from a collection of his preferred music or recordings.	• *D* selects a song or *D* does not.
• Play the song *D* selected.	• *D* attentively listens to music or *D* does not.
• Ask *D* open-ended questions to elicit participation in discussion (e.g., a question that requires a response other than "yes" or "no.")	• *D* answers question or *D* does not.

During the course of treatment, the following was used to chart *D's* progress.

Music Therapy Progress Report Chart

Name of Agency: <u>Custer County Mental Health Center</u>

Patient Name: <u>D</u>   Therapist Name: *John Doe, MT-BC*

Specify goal and objective being worked on in the space provided. Place the appropriate evaluation code under the session date to indicate whether or not the objective was met, if the patient or therapist was absent, or if there was insufficient time to work on the objective. Write a session/ monthly progress report.

Goal #1: <u>D will demonstrate socialization skills by 2-01-96.</u>
Objective #1.1: <u>During music listening, D will verbalize more than a yes or no response in discussion of selected music, in 4 out of 5 sessions by 11-30-95.</u>

Date: *November 1995 / 11-2 / 11-9 / 11-16 / 11-23 / 11-30 /*
Progress: –   P   A   +   +

EVALUATION:
Record a "+" for completion of objective.
Record a "P" for progress toward meeting the objective.
Record a "–" for not meeting objective.
Record an "A" for patient or therapist being absent
Record an "0" for insufficient time during the session to work on the objective.

Session Progress Report/Comments

11-2: D was unresponsive, making no comments.
11-9: Although the objective was not met, D is making progress. He responded with an occasional "yes" or "no" or a nonverbal gesture such as a shrug of the shoulders.
11-16: Therapist was absent — attended NAMT Conference.
11-23: D answered questions about the musical characteristics of the songs (e.g., tempo) using whole sentences.
11-30: D continued discussing songs; it is recommended that two more sessions be conducted to meet the criterion.

Music Therapy Progress Report Chart

Name of Agency: <u>Custer County Mental Health Center</u>

Patient Name: <u>D</u> Therapist Name: *John Doe, MT-BC*

Specify goal and objective being worked on in the space provided. Place the appropriate evaluation code under the session date to indicate whether or not the objective was met, if the patient or therapist was absent, or if there was insufficient time to work on the objective. Write a progress report for each session.

Goal #1: <u>D will demonstrate socialization skills by 2-01-96.</u>
Objective #1.2: <u>During music listening, D will spontaneously verbalize more than a yes or no response in discussion of selected music, in 4 out of 5 sessions by 1-5-96.</u>

Date: *December 1995 / 12-6 / 12-13 / 12-20 / 12-27 /*
Progress: –   P   +   A

EVALUATION:
Record a "+" for completion of objective.
Record a "P" for progress toward meeting the objective.
Record a "–" for not meeting objective.
Record an "A" for patient or therapist being absent
Record an "0" for insufficient time during the session to work on the objective.

Session Progress Report/Comments

12-6: D answered only when prompted.

12-13: D's interest seems to be increasing as he verbalized freely when prompted.

12-20: D spontaneously asked if Bill Haley had died with Buddy Holly. Another patient assured D that he had not, but that the Big Bopper and Richie Valens had died in the airplane crash. D then spontaneously asked to hear some music by the Big Bopper.

12-27: D was absent because he was being seen by the hospital physician.

Case Examples: Adolescence

The following case material provides examples of how to derive multimodal analyses, goals, objectives, and implementation strategies for adolescents.

Case of *M*

DATE: September 17, 1995

M is a 15-year-old male adolescent presently living at a specialized community home. *M* was placed in DHS (Department of Human Services) custody December 3, 1993. Since that time he has spent approximately six weeks living at home with his family. During the rest of the time, he has resided in a variety of different settings including foster care and youth shelter.

M has not had contact with his natural father since he was five months old. His mother was married to an abusive man from 1981–1984. Both mother and child were physically abused. *M*'s abusive stepfather works on an oil rig and his mother is a nurse. *M* has a brother age 17, and a 12-year-old sister.

The *Minnesota Multiphasic Personality Inventory* for adolescents suggests a valid profile. *M*'s pattern of evaluations on the basic clinical scales were similar to adolescents who are referred to treatment because of defiant, impulsive, and mischievous behavior. Their chief defense mechanism is acting out. They are described as assertive, hardheaded, impatient, impulsive, pleasure seeking, good-natured, self-centered, demanding and reckless. *M* showed evidence of an overall low functioning level, a conduct disorder, and some adjustment problems connected to family stresses and the recent change in placement and schools.

M received a psychological evaluation on May 6, 1995. The *Wechsler Intelligence Scale for Children III* indicated *M* to have a verbal IQ of 76, a performance IQ of 79, and a full scale IQ of 76. An October 1993 psychological evaluation however, indicated *M*'s full scale IQ to be 91.

M is reported to have suicidal tendencies. He does not interact well in groups unless he is engaged in sports, in which case he is outspoken. He has been described as having a sociopathic personality, however, his age disqualifies him from such a diagnosis.

After reviewing *M*'s case history and administering the PMTQ for adolescents, the following BASIC I.D. was compiled to provide an overview of *M*'s problems.

BASIC I.D.

MODALITY	PROBLEMS
Behavior	——
Affect	Anger or rage towards others Excessive anxiety Impulsive Difficulty sharing feelings about significant life experiences
Sensation	——
Imagery	——

Cognitive	Lacks problem solving skills Low frustration tolerance Fighting with parents; poor conflict resolution skills.
Interpersonal	Uncooperative behavior Lacks awareness of self and others (e.g., calls others derogatory names)
Drugs	——

Following construction of the above BASIC I.D., *M's* Multimodal Music Therapy Profile was constructed.

Multimodal Music Therapy Profile: *M*

I. MUSIC PREFERENCES

M's favorite type of music is rap. He also likes country and rock. Neutral responses were given in the areas of popular and jazz music. He dislikes religious music and folk music. *M's* favorite group is Criss Cross. *M* indicated he would like to learn to play the guitar.

II. MULTIMODAL PROBLEM ANALYSIS

Affect	Problem	Music Therapy Intervention
A-2	**Exhibits anger or rage towards other people**	• Have the patient select a song from an album to express the anger being felt. Follow by having the patient identify personal, appropriate alternatives for ventilating the anger.
A-4	Excessive anxiety	• Progressive muscle relaxation (PMR). • Guided Imagery – Imagine anxious situations then a positive outcome; follow with discussion. Assign the patient to do imagery and help select appropriate music.
A-5	Impulsive	• Use relaxation techniques such as biofeedback, music response, and key word response. • Give piano or guitar instruction to provide experience at self-control. • Provide for positive peer experiences through music.
A-6	**Difficulty sharing feelings about significant life experiences (e.g., traumas or fears)**	• Music listening with discussion of lyrics related to patient's traumas or fears. • Establish patient trust in the therapist using song writing and improvisational activities.

Interpersonal	Problem	Music Therapy Intervention
IS-1	Uncooperative Behavior	• Involve patient in an instrumental group; assign responsibilities so each patient's cooperation is dependent upon group success, e.g., group improvisation.

| IS-2 | Lacks awareness of self and others (e.g., calls others derogatory names) | • Have the patient accompany other patients, and to take solos while being accompanied in the above group. Encourage other awareness during follow-up discussions, e.g., "I like the way *John* played." |
| IS-3 | Withdrawal (e.g., does not talk when in a group) | • Encourage group involvement by utilizing activities of interest to the patient, such as music listening with graded discussion, music composition, instrumental, group singing, and musical games. |

Cognitive	Problem	Music Therapy Intervention
C-2	**Lacks problem solving skills**	• Use guided imagery and music relaxation. During guided imagery ask the patient to imagine problem situations and to mentally rehearse being in control. In follow-up discussion, give patient experience at discovering successful management strategies for problems.
C-3	**Low frustration tolerance**	• Adjust above guitar or piano lessons to insure success, with the goal of increasing frustration tolerance. • Involve the patient in additional activities such as song writing and music improvisation to reduce frustration and inappropriate behavior.
C-8 through C-10	**Fighting with parents; Poor conflict resolution skills**	• Improvisation using instruments to represent family members; discuss appropriate solutions. • Discuss appropriate solutions to problem oriented song lyrics (e.g., "Cat's in the Cradle.") Generalize to patient.

III. POST INTERVIEW OBSERVATIONS

Post interview observations indicated a high degree of concentration, retention, and an adequate attention span. *M* exhibited appropriate facial expressions, posture, and was appropriately groomed.

The above initial assessment indicated *M* to have Affective, Interpersonal, and Cognitive problems. In addition, they are the types of problems most frequently treated by music therapists. Although additional problems may be noted later during the treatment phase, the above initial assessment provides information concerning the most important problems, and ample data for initiating a music therapy program of treatment, complete with music therapy goals and objectives. *M* therefore, was accepted for music therapy.

The intervention plans and strategies designed for *M* contain goals, behavioral objectives, procedures, and evaluation criteria. Following is an example of an intervention plan for helping *M* to appropriately express his anger.

MUSIC THERAPY INTERVENTION PLAN

NAME: *M*   CASE NO: <u>0002</u>

DATE OF ASSESSMENT: <u>10-02-95</u>

Music Therapy Goals and Objectives

Goal #1: <u>Affect-Anger</u>

Goal Statement: <u>*M* will learn appropriate methods of expressing anger by 1-2-96.</u>

Objective #1.1 Objective Statement: <u>During music listening, *M* will select songs expressing anger</u> <u>to which he relates in 4 out of 5 sessions by 12-01-95.</u>

Person Responsible: *John Doe, MT-BC*

Date Started: <u>10-09-95</u>   Date Ended: _____

Reason Ended: _____

Objective #1.2 Objective Statement: <u>In discussions that follow music listening, *M* will verbalize</u> <u>5 personal, appropriate alternatives for ventilating his anger in 4 out of 5 sessions by 1-2-96.</u>

Person Responsible: *John Doe, MT-BC*

Date Started: <u>10-09-95</u>   Date Ended: _____

Reason Ended: _____

Objective #1.3 Objective Statement: <u>[NOTE: Write any additional objectives for Goal #1 here.]</u>

Person Responsible: _____

Date Started: _____   Date Ended: _____

Reason Ended: _____

Following construction of the intervention plan, the implementation strategy is constructed. Following is an example of an implementation strategy constructed for *M*.

IMPLEMENTATION STRATEGY

NAME: *M*   CASE NO: 0002

DATE OF ASSESSMENT: 10-02-95

Objective #1.1: During music listening, *M* will select songs expressing anger to which he relates in 4 out of 5 sessions 12 by 12-01-95.

Materials Needed: Guitar or piano, psychiatric song or lyric book.

Reinforcement Schedule: Continuous verbal reinforcement in sessions 1–10.

THERAPIST BEHAVIOR	PATIENT BEHAVIOR
• Prompt *M* to select a song that describes his feelings.	• *M* selects a song or *M* does not.
• Play the song for *M*.	
• Ask *M* why he chose the song.	• *M* gives reason or *M* does not.
• Ask *M*, "What feelings does the song describe?"	• *M* gives describes feelings in song or *M* does not.
• Follow in discussion.	• If *M* does not select a song expressing his anger, repeat the above procedure except ask him to select a song expressing his anger.

Following the construction of the Implementation Strategy, music therapy sessions were initiated and the following chart was used to record *M's* progress.

Music Therapy Progress Report Chart

Name of Agency: <u>Custer County Mental Health Center</u>

Patient Name: <u>M</u>   Therapist Name: *John Doe, MT-BC*

Specify goal and objective being worked on in the space provided. Place the appropriate evaluation code under the session date to indicate whether or not the objective was met, if the patient or therapist was absent, or if there was insufficient time to work on the objective. Write a progress report for each session.

Goal #1: <u>M will learn appropriate methods of expressing anger by 1-02-96.</u>
Objective #1.1: <u>During music listening, M will select songs expressing anger to which he relates, in 4 out of 5 sessions by 12-01-95.</u>

Date: *October 1995*   / 10-9 / 10-16 / 10-23 / 10-30 /
Progress: –   P   –   +

EVALUATION:
Record a "+" for completion of objective.
Record a "P" for progress toward meeting the objective.
Record a "–" for not meeting objective.
Record an "A" for patient or therapist being absent
Record an "0" for insufficient time during the session to work on the objective.

Session Progress Report/Comments

_____

_____

_____

_____

_____

_____

_____

_____

_____

_____

Music Therapy Progress Report Chart

Name of Agency: <u>Custer County Mental Health Center</u>

Patient Name: <u>M</u>   Therapist Name: *John Doe, MT-BC*

Specify goal and objective being worked on in the space provided. Place the appropriate evaluation code under the session date to indicate whether or not the objective was met, if the patient or therapist was absent, or if there was insufficient time to work on the objective. Write a progress report for each session.

Goal #1: <u>M will learn appropriate methods of expressing anger by 1-02-96.</u>
Objective #1.2: <u>In discussions that follow music listening, M will verbalize 5 personal,</u>
<u>appropriate alternatives for ventilating his anger in 4 out of 5 sessions by 1-2-96.</u>

Date: *October 1995*   / 10-9 / 10-16 / 10-23 / 10-30 /
Progress: A   –   P   +

EVALUATION:
Record a "+" for completion of objective.
Record a "P" for progress toward meeting the objective.
Record a "–" for not meeting objective.
Record an "A" for patient or therapist being absent
Record an "0" for insufficient time during the session to work on the objective.

Session Progress Report/Comments

_____

_____

_____

_____

_____

_____

_____

_____

_____

_____

The case of *B* provides a further example of how to construct a multimodal music therapy profile for adolescents.

Case of *B*

Date: September 24, 1995

B is a 16-year-old male adolescent presently living at a specialized community home. *B* was placed in DHS custody May 15, 1993. Since that time *B* has resided in a variety of different settings including foster care and youth shelter.

B's biological father is reported to be in prison. *B* was made aware of his identity a year and a half ago, but has never met him. *B's* mother was using drugs at the time of his birth, and his great grandparents requested and received custodial care of him at three months. His natural mother and stepfather visit him sporadically. Contact with siblings is minimal and inconsistent.

B was born chemically dependent. At age three, *B* was diagnosed as being hyperactive and placed on Ritalin. He continued this medication until he was in kindergarten.

B received a psychological evaluation in 1995. The *Wechsler Intelligence Scale-Revised* indicated *B* to have a verbal IQ of 80, a performance IQ of 101, and a full scale IQ of 89. His strength was his ability to organize and remember visually perceived material as well as visual motor coordination. Weaknesses included verbal comprehension, difficulty with concentration, and a tendency to be distractive. The *Bender Gestalt* indicated developmental lags, and immature mental and emotional development. Feelings of inferiority and the tendency to withdraw from others were revealed, along with hostile feelings of a covert nature. Projective drawings indicated emotional impulsive desires to repress thoughts and memories with an almost childlike avoidance of reality. *B* makes attempts at controlling his emotions but few resources render him successful.

After reviewing *B's* case history and administering the PMTQ for adolescents, the following BASIC I.D. was compiled.

BASIC I.D.

MODALITY	PROBLEMS
Behavior	Mediocre attention span and concentration Inadequate eye contact
Affect	Excessive anxiety Difficulty relating life experiences to others Observe for signs of emotional immaturity
Sensation	——
Imagery	——
Cognitive	Weakness in verbal comprehension Feelings of inferiority
Interpersonal	Withdrawn Does not engage in leisure activities May lack knowledge of leisure activities
Drugs	——

Following construction of the above BASIC I.D., *B's* Multimodal Music Therapy Profile was constructed.

Multimodal Music Therapy Profile: *B*

I. MUSIC PREFERENCES

B stated he likes country, popular, rock, and religious music equally. He is neutral about jazz and dislikes folk music. *B's* favorite group is Alice in Chains. *B* expressed a desire to participate in a music listening group.

II. MULTIMODAL PROBLEM ANALYSIS

Affect	Problem	Music Therapy Intervention
A-4	Excessive anxiety	• Progressive muscle relaxation. • Guided imagery – imagine anxious situations then a positive outcome; discuss. Assign the patient to do imagery and assist in selecting appropriate music.
A-6	Difficulty relating life experiences to others	• Establish patient trust in the music therapist. Use song writing, improvisation, and song lyric discussion related to the patient's fears or traumas.

Interpersonal	Problem	Music Therapy Intervention
IS-3	Withdrawal	• Encourage group involvement by utilizing activities of interest to the patient, such as music listening with graded discussion, music composition, instrumental, group singing, and musical games.
IS-4 through IS-5	May lack knowledge of leisure activities. Does not engage in leisure activities	• Give music lessons; encourage home practice. • Consider patient involvement in music groups such as school or community band, orchestra, chorus, church choir, and popular music ensemble. • Expose patient to arts entertainment and activities in the community.

Behavior	Problem	Music Therapy Intervention
B-2	Mediocre attention span and concentration	• Adjust involvement in music lessons to accommodate attention span (e.g., length of lesson and practice time, five minute breaks during practice time, gradually longer playing times).
Not specified	Inadequate eye contact	• Gradually encourage more and more eye contact from the patient during the above music therapy activities. Require the patient to watch for musical cues.

III. POST INTERVIEW OBSERVATIONS

Post interview impressions indicate a mediocre degree of concentration, retention, and attention span. *B* exhibited appropriate facial expressions and posture, and was groomed properly. Eye contact appeared to be inadequate.

B's profile indicates eye contact as a problem. Although eye contact is not listed in the manual under Adolescents, it was listed as a problem in *B's* profile because of his inadequate eye contact during the initial interview.

The above initial assessment indicated *B* to have affective, interpersonal, and behavioral problems. Other problems across the BASIC I.D. may emerge during treatment, especially if the music therapist decides to perform a second order BASIC I.D. as described in Chapter 1. The above profile however, provides ample justification and information for the initiation of music therapy with *B*. The decision therefore, was to accept *B* for music therapy.

Case Example: Childhood
Following is an example of an initial assessment with *J*.

Case of *J*

Date: September 22, 1995

J is a six-year-old female who has been receiving treatment at a community mental health center since July 29, 1995. *J's* mother and father have been divorced for 18 months, and were separated for four years before the divorce. *J's* mother has since remarried. *J* has a sister age four, and an 18-month-old brother. *J* is presently living at home with her mother and stepfather. *J's* biological father, who is homosexual and living with another man, sees *J* every other week.

In kindergarten *J* is learning slowly and has difficulty recalling concepts. *J* likes to read books, listen to music, and play with dolls in her spare time. *J's* mother reported that *J* frequently wets the bed. *J* frequently states "I want to be myself; nobody loves me." *J* was thought to be autistic at an earlier age. She was reported to engage in seductive behavior and sexual play that could be the result of overstimulation through overexposure to sexual material. No definite incidence of sexual abuse was noted.

During *J's* personal interview she was very talkative and engaged in a great deal of story telling. During the interview she exhibited an unusual tremor in the upper part of her body. Despite the unusual body movements and apparent learning difficulties, *J* appeared intelligent in some areas. No physical developmental delays were noted.

J's problems were not interacting well with peers, learning problems, poor emotional expression, and unprovoked violent, angry behavior. Her strengths were that her mother and stepfather are supportive, she is enrolled in kindergarten, and her mother adequately takes care of her needs. *J* was referred for a neurological examination and admitted to group therapy, with individual therapy provided as needed. *J's* mother was referred to outpatient therapy. *J* was given the following diagnosis:

Axis I: 309.28   Adjustment Disorder With Mixed Anxiety and Depressed Mood.
           V61.20   Parent-Child Relational Problem.
           299.80   Pervasive Developmental Disorder NOS
Axis II: None
Axis III: None
Axis IV: Separation and divorce of parents; remarriage of mother.
Axis V: Current GAF: 50

After interviewing J's mother, observing J, reading the assessments of other professionals, and administering the PMTQ for children to J's mother, the following BASIC I.D. was constructed for J.

BASIC I.D.

MODALITY	PROBLEMS
Behavior	Unassertive, does not express needs Off task, easily distracted, poor concentration, short attention span Hits peers Poor eye contact
Affect	Has trouble describing how others feel Exhibits too many emotional extremes
Sensation	
Imagery	
Cognitive	Difficulty following directions Makes negative self statements, low self-esteem, lacks self-confidence to participate in group activities Poor method and quality of approach to tasks Makes derogatory comments to peers if they don't do what she wants
Interpersonal	Does not follow rules and regulations Makes negative comments to peers (i.e., name calling) Minimal or no verbal interaction with peers Is not attentive in structured activities (e.g., does not pay attention to others) Poor leadership skills
Drugs	Poor speech articulation Poor comprehension

Following construction of the above BASIC I.D., J's Multimodal Music Therapy Profile was constructed.

Multimodal Music Therapy Profile: *J*

I. MUSIC PREFERENCES

J's mother stated J strongly prefers popular, children's, folk, religious, new age, and classical music. She likes country music and is neutral about rock music. Her favorite recording is Kitaro (New Age).

II. MULTIMODAL PROBLEM ANALYSIS

Interpersonal	Problem	Music Therapy Intervention
IS-1	Does not follow rules and regulations	• Use contingent music techniques.
IS-1	Makes negative comments to peers (i.e., name calling)	• Use contingent music techniques.
IS-2	Minimal or no verbal interaction with peers	• Use a rhythm band to encourage nonverbal peer interaction. • Use music listening techniques in which patient chooses songs for peer, or that describes peer. • Encourage interaction in a variety of "fun" music activities.
IS-5	Is not attentive in structured activities (e.g., does not pay attention to others)	• During a pentatonic instrumental ensemble, use eye contact to cue or communicate when each individual is to start or stop playing her instrument. Reinforce on task behavior.
IS-7	Poor leadership skills	• Assign the patient leadership roles during the above rhythm instrument activity (e.g., display STOP and GO signs to signal when the group starts or stops playing).

Behavior	Problem	Music Therapy Intervention
B-1	Unassertive; does not express needs	• Have patient conduct above instrumental groups with a baton communicating dynamics, tempo, starting and stopping. • Elicit nonverbal and verbal choice of instrument. • Play musical games that require the patient to ask questions.
B-2	**Off task, easily distracted, poor concentration, short attention span**	• Reinforce in seat behavior using instrumental play activities. • Have patient sing while maintaining a rhythmic beat; use gradually longer songs.
B-4	Hits peers.	• Involve the patient in a puppet show focused on a musical drama about feelings. • Contingent music.
B-5	**Poor eye contact**	• Elicit eye contact by singing the child's name in a song. • Have patient give and receive performance cues using eye contact in above instrumental activities.

Drugs (Motor)	Problem	Music Therapy Intervention
D-2.4	Poor speech articulation	• Emphasize clear pronunciation while singing songs and chanting the lyrics. Review speech pathology assessment.
D-2.5	Poor comprehension	• Discuss the meaning of song lyrics during the above singing activities.

Cognitive	Problem	Music Therapy Intervention
C-1	**Difficulty following directions**	• Assign tasks during above instrumental activities (e.g., playing an ostinato rhythmic pattern). • Give directions during above singing activities (e.g., finding page numbers). • Use body action songs and simple dances requiring the following of one-step, two-step, and multistep directions.
C-3	**Makes negative self statements, low self-esteem, lacks self-confidence to participate in group activities**	• Record number of positive self and peer statements as patient assesses musical accomplishments. • Increase self-confidence through successful group participation (e.g., above instrumental groups; games such as "Music Charades").
C-4	Poor method and quality of approach to tasks	• Instrumental performance activities (e.g., using the autoharp to provide a chordal accompaniment to a song; playing an ostinato pattern on the marimba.)
C-5	Makes derogatory comments to peers if they don't do what she wants	• During song writing, teach the sharing of concepts by singing the children's thoughts, feelings, and ideas about appropriate ways of meeting one's needs.

Affect	Problem	Music Therapy Intervention
A-1	Has trouble describing how others feel, exhibits too many emotional extremes	• Teach patient to describe and to appropriately express feelings. (e.g., see "feeling card" activity, instrumental, and song techniques in the manual).

III. POST INTERVIEW OBSERVATIONS

J exhibited poor eye contact, limited concentration, and short attention span. Interpersonal relationships appeared mediocre. She seems very interested in music.

J's PMTQ results indicated deficits in telling time, counting money, memorizing the letters of the alphabet, and counting. Although these deficits were rated a "5" in the PMTQ, they were not given top priority in J's music therapy plan. Because of the developmental level of the patient (CA = 6) and the severity of J's emotional problems, top priority was assigned to treating the emotional problems. Plans were made however, to meet with J's teacher to discuss academic goals.

Because J had a multitude of the types of problems music therapists commonly treat, J was accepted for music therapy.

Following is J's Music Therapy Intervention Plan for improving her ability to follow directions.

MUSIC THERAPY INTERVENTION PLAN

NAME: *J*_____   CASE NO: <u>0004</u>
DATE OF ASSESSMENT: <u>9-22-95</u>_____

Music Therapy Goals and Objectives

Goal #1: <u>Cognitive-Following Directions</u>_____
Goal Statement: <u>*J* will follow directions in group activities by 10-23-95.</u>_____

Objective #1.1 Objective Statement: <u>During an instrumental activity, *J* will play her instrument</u> <u>when her instrument and name are mentioned in a song selected by the therapist, 4 out of</u> <u>5 times correctly.</u>_____
Person Responsible: *Jane Doe, MT-BC*_____
Date Started: <u>10-02-95</u>_____   Date Ended: _____
Reason Ended: _____

Objective #1.2 Objective Statement: <u>During group activity, *J* will verbally select a song that the</u> <u>person sitting next to her might enjoy, one song per session, for one consecutive month.</u>

Person Responsible: *Jane Doe, MT-BC*_____
Date Started: <u>10-02-95</u>_____   Date Ended: _____
Reason Ended: _____

Objective #1.3 Objective Statement: <u>[NOTE: Write any additional objectives for Goal #1 here.]</u>

Person Responsible: _____
Date Started: _____   Date Ended: _____
Reason Ended: _____

Following is *J's* implementation strategy for improving her ability to follow directions.

IMPLEMENTATION STRATEGY

NAME: *J*   CASE NO: 0004

DATE OF ASSESSMENT: 9-22-95

Objective #1.1: During an instrumental activity, *J* will play her instrument when her instrument and name are mentioned in a song selected by the therapist, 4 out of 5 times correctly.

Materials Needed: Rhythm instruments, guitar, or piano.

Reinforcement Schedule: Contingent music; continuous positive reinforcement.

THERAPIST BEHAVIOR	PATIENT BEHAVIOR
• Ask all the children to join hands with each other (to form a circle).	• Child joins hands or child does not.
• Seat the children "Indian style" and give each child a rhythm instrument	• Child sits on the floor or child does not.
	• Child appropriately accepts or rejects rhythm instrument or child inappropriately accepts or rejects rhythm instrument.*
	(*If child makes a negative comment while being handed her instrument, tell the child that is not the appropriate way to disagree; assist the child in appropriately disagreeing. Either do not give the child an instrument and explain why, or give the child an instrument if the child makes a satisfactory disagreement.)
• Explain to the children that you (the therapist) are going to sing a song and in the song their names and their instruments are mentioned. When they hear their instrument and name they play until another instrument starts. Explain to the children that if they play out of turn they will be asked to sit out one turn in the song.	
	•Child plays when her name and name of instrument are sung or child does not.

The following chart was used to record *J's* progress.

Music Therapy Progress Report Chart

Name of Agency: <u>Custer County Mental Health Center</u>

Patient Name: <u>J</u>   Therapist Name: *Jane Doe, MT-BC*

Specify goal and objective being worked on in the space provided. Place the appropriate evaluation code under the session date to indicate whether or not the objective was met, if the patient or therapist was absent, or if there was insufficient time to work on the objective. Write a progress report for each session.

Goal #1: <u>J will follow directions in group activities by 10-23-95.</u>
Objective #1.1: <u>During an instrumental activity, J will play her instrument when her instrument and name are mentioned in a song selected by the therapist, 4 out of 5 times correctly by 10-23-95.</u>

Date: *October 1995*   / 10-1 / 10-7 / 10-14 / 10-21 / 10-28 /
Progress: –   P   +   A   +

EVALUATION:
Record a "+" for completion of objective.
Record a "P" for progress toward meeting the objective.
Record a "–" for not meeting objective.
Record an "A" for patient or therapist being absent
Record an "0" for insufficient time during the session to work on the objective.

Session Progress Report/Comments

_____

_____

_____

_____

_____

_____

_____

_____

_____

_____

Music Therapy Progress Report Chart

Name of Agency: <u>Custer County Mental Health Center</u>

Patient Name: <u>J</u>   Therapist Name: *Jane Doe, MT-BC*

Specify goal and objective being worked on in the space provided. Place the appropriate evaluation code under the session date to indicate whether or not the objective was met, if the patient or therapist was absent, or if there was insufficient time to work on the objective. Write a progress report for each session.

Goal #1: <u>J will follow directions in group activities by 10-23-95.</u>
Objective #1.2: <u>During group activity, J will verbally select a song that the person sitting next to her might enjoy, one song per session, for one consecutive month by 10-23-95.</u>

Date: *October 1995*   / 10-1 / 10-7 / 10-14 / 10-21 / 10-28 /
Progress: –   –   +   +   +

EVALUATION:
Record a "+" for completion of objective.
Record a "P" for progress toward meeting the objective.
Record a "–" for not meeting objective.
Record an "A" for patient or therapist being absent
Record an "0" for insufficient time during the session to work on the objective.

Session Progress Report/Comments

_____

_____

_____

_____

_____

_____

_____

_____

_____

_____

Following is a summary of the seven-stage multimodal music therapy process:
1. Review the patient's case history and other assessment information (if available).
2. Administer the PMTQ that is appropriate for the patient's chronological age level.
3. Construct a BASIC I.D.
4. Construct a Multimodal Music Therapy Profile that is appropriate for the patient's chronological age level.
5. Write one Music Therapy Intervention Plan for each goal.
6. Write one Music Therapy Implementation Strategy for each objective.
7. Complete one Music Therapy Progress Report Chart for each objective.

Alternate Strategies for Documenting Intervention and Progress

The recording format prescribed in the Music Therapy Intervention Plan and the Music Therapy Progress Report Chart is most useful when the therapist has few goals and wishes to illustrate progress toward achieving single objectives over time. However, as the number of goals and objectives increase, the amount of paperwork required to use the above format also increases, reducing the manageability of the model. The following recording format, illustrated with the case of Mark, may be used in situations where it is necessary to maintain and document progress toward numerous music therapy goals and objectives written for a single patient.

Mark, age four, had profound global developmental delay. Mark's level of functioning on standardized tests measuring various types of adaptive behavior ranged from a low of six months to a high of one year two months. After assessing Mark, the music therapist wrote the following "Individualized Intervention Plan." Note the intervention plan used for Mark contains four goals, eliminating the need to have a separate page for each goal as with other intervention plans in this book. Another feature of Mark's intervention plan is that it provides space for parental input and requests his parent's signature. This procedure of requesting parental input and a signature is recommended for music therapists in private practice, and commonly followed in institutional treatment plans or Individualized Educational Programs for children. A blank copy of the Individualized Intervention Plan has been placed in Appendix IV as an alternate recording form.

Name of Agency: <u>Therapeutic Directions in Music</u>

Patient Name: <u>Mark</u>   Date: <u>April 30, 1998</u>

Therapist Name: <u>*Jane Doe, MT-BC*</u>

INDIVIDUALIZED INTERVENTION PLAN

Long-Term Goal #1: <u>To improve ability to follow simple commands and fine motor control.</u>

Short-Term Objective #1.1: <u>When given a command in a song such as putting an item in a bag, box, etc., or removing an item from a bag or box, Mark will follow the command three out of four times for four consecutive sessions.</u>

Short-Term Objective #1.2: <u>When given commands in a song to start and stop playing instruments such as the drum and bells, Mark will start and stop playing on verbal cue without requiring physical prompting for three out of four trials over three consecutive sessions.</u>

Long-Term Goal #2: To increase simple communication skills through signing and singing one syllable sounds.

Short-Term Objective #2.1: Mark will sign four out of six words correctly when he is asked for them in a song presentation for three consecutive sessions.

Short-Term Objective #2.2: Mark will sign two syllables four consecutive times when the syllable is presented in a song format for three consecutive sessions.

Long-Term Goal #3: To improve body awareness and awareness of others.

Short-Term Objective #3.1: When presented with songs that request Mark to identify body parts, he will identify four out of seven body parts for four consecutive sessions.

Short-Term Objective #3.2: During music therapy activities Mark will maintain eye contact with the therapist for the duration of one song with verbal prompting for four consecutive sessions.

Long-Term Goal #4: To improve gross motor movement.

Short-Term Objective #4.1: Mark will follow movements presented in a song such as standing up, walking, clapping hands, and swaying with verbal prompting only at least one time for four consecutive sessions.

PLAN: Mark will attend music therapy sessions at the Therapeutic Directions clinic independently if possible. Session frequency shall be one time per week for 50–60 minutes. During the session, the patient will participate in a variety of music therapy activities designed to be pleasurable yet meet the objectives written above.

Parent Response to Intervention Plan: *The goals and objectives in this plan correspond with those in Mark's IEP at school. I am in agreement with this plan and will reinforce the plan's goals and objectives at home.*

I am in agreement with this plan, and agree to attend sessions regularly to allow for optimal benefit. If I must cancel a session, I agree to give advanced notice if possible.

SIGNATURES:

Janet Smith
Parent

Jane Doe, MT-BC
Therapist

The final form titled "Session Progress Note" was used to record the progress Mark made toward the goals and objectives listed in his intervention plan. The Session Progress Note is similar to the Music Therapy Progress Report Chart discussed earlier in this book in that the purpose of both is to record progress toward achieving goals and objectives. The two formats differ in that the former is for reporting progress toward *numerous goals and objectives for a single session*, whereas the latter is used for reporting progress toward a *single objective for numerous sessions*. Hence, the two forms serve similar but opposite purposes.

A Session Progress Note contains the following information as illustrated below:
1. Title of the facility (e.g., Therapeutic Directions in Music)
2. The name of the therapist
3. The title of the form (SESSION PROGRESS NOTE)
4. The date of the session (e.g., 5/24/98)
5. The length and time of the session (e.g., 60 min./0900–1000)
6. A session summary (e.g., Mark attended session this date...)
7. The number of the objective being evaluated (e.g., 1.1) as listed in the Intervention Plan.
8. An evaluation code chosen from the following:
   Record a "+" for completion of objective.
   Record a "P" for progress toward meeting the objective.
   Record a "–" for not meeting objective.
   Record an "A" for patient or therapist being absent
   Record an "0" for insufficient time during the session to work on the objective.
9. Following the evaluation code, a comment which often relates to patient performance of the objective, whether the objective will be continued, etc.

A blank copy of the Session Progress Note has been placed in Appendix IV as an alternate recording form.

Name of Agency: <u>Therapeutic Directions in Music</u>

Patient Name: <u>Mark</u>   Therapist Name: *Jane Doe, MT-BC*

SESSION PROGRESS NOTE

5/24/98 (60min./0900–1000) Mark attended session this date at the Therapeutic Directions clinic. He seemed eager to come in and begin the music. When his mother told him she had to go he reached up and gave her a big kiss and then got on the floor. He first went over to the piano. Mark's mother had reported that on one occasion he played the piano at home for a full 25 minutes without diverting his attention. During this session, Mark tolerated all the activities well. He did not have any incidences of expressing frustration or agitation. He was more distractible than in the previous session, and seemed to be interested in exploration. On three occasions he had to be redirected back to the therapy room.

1.1: (P)   Mark dropped two items in the box today with physical prompting by the therapist placing her hand over the box and lightly shaking her arm. He was given much praise. Will continue with this objective.
1.2: (–)   Mark did not seem focused on this activity. He played the drum one time independently and then seemed more focused on self-stimulating behavior. He also did not seem focused on playing the bells. He had to be encouraged several times and even then played only for a few seconds. Will continue with this objective.

2.1: (–)   Mark waved hello with physical and verbal prompting. He did not wave good-bye. The signing intervention which includes other signs was not addressed this date. Will continue with this objective.

2.2: (P)   Mark attended well to the singing activities this date. When presented with the horse and the animal sound for horse, he made the sound "errr." Praise was given. This was the only syllable he stated during the two songs presented, however, after this he seemed more vocal and began to make sounds himself which he frequently uses (e.g., ahta, keekee).

3.1: (P)   Mark demonstrated eagerness to look into the mirror during this intervention and attended to this activity for a great length of time. He voluntarily touched his ears when the therapist sang for him to touch his nose, however, he was praised for touching a body part. He touched her ears again when the therapist requested him to touch his hair. This is the second time he has voluntarily touched a body part on command even if it wasn't the correct one. He allowed the therapist to assist him without *resistance*.

3.2: (P)   Mark demonstrated improved eye contact by looking at the therapist more frequently, but did so in intervals rather than for the length of a song. He seemed more alert and responsive. Will continue with this objective.

4.1 (P)   Mark continues to follow movements with physical prompting. His interest in exploring was used as time to practice physical movement, especially walking. He was willing to walk with less assistance.

Reliability and Validity of the PMTQ

The PMTQ may be considered a behavioral interview questionnaire. Since the aims, assumptions, and applications of behavioral assessment differ from those of traditional assessment, issues such as reliability, validity, standardization, and normalization are a matter of controversy. For example, from a behavioral assessment perspective, the validity of the PMTQ is dependent upon how accurate the individual patient is at reporting her problems. Reliability is dependent upon how accurately the interviewer records the patient's problems. Also, poor test-retest is more likely to be due to variance in the environmental conditions than in the data collection procedure (Groth-Marnat, 1990). In addition, traditional reliability and validity estimates calculated from group scores or means report group performance rather than individual performance. Reliability and validity based on group data, as well as normative comparisons, are frequently viewed by behavioral assessment advocates as both irrelevant and inappropriate since they believe reliability and validity is only important in so far as it pertains to the performance of the individual (Groth-Marnat, 1990).

Standardization is another area of controversy. Standardization attempts to set the testing procedure so the test is administered the same way to all examinees. Standardization is very important if the examinee's score is to be meaningfully compared with the scores of his or her peers (*inter-individual* comparisons). The primary purpose of the PMTQ however, is to pinpoint the individual's problems (*intra-individual* comparisons) rather than to compare the individual's problems with those of his or her peers. When administering the *Wechsler Intelligence Scale* for example, the examiner is not allowed to explain, clarify, or interpret the test items in his own words for the examinee, but instead must follow the set testing procedure specified in the Wechsler manual. In the case of the PMTQ, occasionally a patient will ask for a clarification, or require an example in order to accurately respond to a PMTQ item. If the PMTQ were standardized like the Wechsler the examiner would be prohibited from doing the above resulting in a loss of information, perhaps critical information, concerning the patient's problems. As indicated in the following paragraphs, the PMTQ test procedure is however, specific enough to insure stability of examinee performance over a period of time. Other behavioral assessment advocates have argued for the use of traditional psychometric techniques in the evaluation of behavioral assessment (Anderson, Cancelli, & Kratochill, 1984; Gresham, 1984). In view of the present controversy, the following paragraphs present psychometric issues relating to the PMTQ from the perspectives of both behavioral and traditional assessment.

Reliability

   Reliability refers to the consistency with which a test measures, or "…the extent to which an experiment, test, or any measuring procedure yields the same results on repeated trials" (Carmines & Zeller, 1979). Blodgett and Davis (1994) investigated the test-retest reliability of the PMTQ with 20 undergraduate university music students. With a three week intervening interval between test and retest the composite reliabilities were Part I: Music, $r_s = .79$; Part II: Multimodal Problem Analysis, $r_s = .90$; and Part III: Post Interview Observations, $r_s = .83$. The reliability estimates for Part II: Multimodal Problem Analysis subtests were Behavior, $r_s = .76$; Cognitive, $r_s = .83$; Affect, $r_s = .82$; Interpersonal, $r_s = .49$; and Drugs, $r_s = .84$. Blodgett and Davis also investigated the inter-scorer reliability of the PMTQ. Inter-scorer reliability indicates the extent two or more examiners will score the test similarly (George, 1980). To test inter-scorer reliability Blodgett and Davis had subjects take the PMTQ twice in immediate succession. Half the subjects were tested by examiner A first and half were tested by examiner B first. The inter-scorer composite reliability estimates were Part I: Music, $r_s = .92$; and Part II: Multimodal Problem Analysis, $r_s = .94$. Results for Part III: Post Interview Observations were not reported. The inter-scorer reliability estimates for Part II: Multimodal Problem Analysis subtests were Behavior, $r_s = .84$; Cognitive, $r_s = .93$; Affect, $r_s = .93$; Interpersonal, $r_s = .50$; and Drugs, $r_s = .76$.

   The test-retest reliabilities of the above subtests were somewhat higher when the PMTQs for adults, adolescents, and children were administered to 12 psychiatric patients of various chronological age levels (or their parents in the case of children) (Murray, 1994). With a three week intervening interval between test and retest, Murray reported composite reliabilities followed by their level of significance as Part I: Music, $r_s = .77$, $p < .01$; Part II: Multimodal Problem Analysis, $r_s = .90$, $p < .001$; and Part III: Post Interview Observations, $r_s = .92$. The reliability estimates and significance levels Murray reported for Part II: Multimodal Problem Analysis subtests were Behavior, $r_s = .90$, $p < .001$; Cognitive, $r_s = .95$, $p < .001$; Affect, $r_s = .97$, $p < .001$; Interpersonal, $r_s = .95$, $p < .001$; and Drugs, $r_s = .94$, $p < .001$.

   The above studies independently indicate the PMTQ has adequate reliability. Carmines and Zeller (1979) have suggested that widely used scales for clinical use should have a reliability of not less than .80. The Interpersonal subtest yielded much higher reliability when administered to Murray's psychiatric patients than when administered to Blodgett's and Davis's university students. A possible reason for Blodgett's and Davis's finding is that the Interpersonal subtest measures predominately state variables rather than trait variables. According to Groth-Marnat (1990), "The practical implication of this is that, if the variable measures a state, then relatively wide fluctuations can be expected and thus the lower test-retest reliabilities would be more acceptable" (102). Stated differently, if the prevailing moods of the university students were different on the second testing, then they may answer the test items differently to coincide with their different moods. A possible reason for the high reliability of the Interpersonal subtest with psychiatric patients is that the mood of most chronic patients may tend to be more stable than that of university students, as in the case of flat affect, or because of mood controlling medication. Because of the pilot nature of the above studies and the encouraging reliability coefficients, further reliability research involving a larger number of subjects is warranted.

Validity

Validity is the extent a test measures what it purports, or claims to measure (Popham, 1978). The PMTQ purports to measure the extent that patients have those problems most commonly treated using music therapy. A crucial factor determining the validity of the PMTQ therefore, would be the extent that patient problems reflected in the PMTQ represent problems music therapists most frequently treat. Stated differently, is the domain of problems in the PMTQ representative of the problems most frequently treated using music therapy?

The PMTQ is similar to a *criterion-referenced test* in that it is a measure of intra-individual differences. More specifically, it references performance to a standard or criterion, rather than to the performance of others, and provides specific information about the needs of the individual (Panell & Laabs, 1979). Unlike criterion-referenced tests, norm-referenced tests such as intelligence tests do not provide information specific enough to enable the practitioner to initiate or design a program of intervention. A good criterion-referenced test provides a specific picture of just what the examinee can or cannot do (Popham, 1978), or in the case of the PMTQ, just what problems the examinee does or does not have in terms of the problems music therapist treat most frequently (the criterion).

It is generally agreed that the type of validity essential and of paramount concern to a criterion-referenced test is *content validity* (Gronlund, 1973; Popham, 1978; Popham & Husek, 1969; Schoenfeldt, Schoenfeld, Acker, & Perlson, 1976; Swezey, 1981). The above question concerning the extent that patient problems reflected in the PMTQ represent problems music therapists most frequently treat would therefore be a question of content validity. Two types of content validity applicable to the PMTQ has been referred to by Popham (1978) as *domain-selection validity* and *descriptive validity*. Domain-selection validity pertains to how the content of the PMTQ was selected, and descriptive validity is the degree to which the test items are congruent with the descriptions in the test manual. In the case of the PMTQ, the degree of congruency would be determined between the test items and the problems in this clinical manual that are listed under Adults, Adolescents, and Children.

Domain selection validity. Multimodal psychiatric music therapy is a data-based model originating from scientific survey methodology. The contents of the PMTQ is based on data derived from the survey. For a complete description of the survey the reader is referred to Cassity and Cassity (1994). Aspects of the survey relating to domain selection validity are as follows:

1. A questionnaire was constructed to obtain the patient problems music therapist assess most frequently. Following construction of the questionnaire, a panel of five registered music therapists employed in AMTA-approved clinical training facilities assessed the clarity of the questionnaire items, the ease with which responses could be provided for the items, and the success of the questionnaire in surveying the topic it was constructed to survey. The panel did not participate in the study other than to judge the questionnaire. Of the five music therapists, four were eclectic and one was of psychodynamic therapeutic philosophy. The four eclectic music therapists agreed the questionnaire was appropriate for the purposes for which it was designed. The psychodynamic music therapist, however, indicated the questionnaire did not relate to her practice of music therapy. Caution must be exercised, therefore, in generalizing the results of the survey, or the PMTQ to psychodynamic settings.

2. The survey population was restricted to clinical training directors (CTDs) partially because CTDs as a group probably are among the most (if not the most) experienced clinicians in the music therapy profession. Limitations have been associated with previous studies that have surveyed music therapy skills and practices without controlling for limited experience among the respondents (Jensen & McKinney, 1990). Popham (1978) also recommends the experience of the judges be considered in establishing domain selection validity.

3. The questionnaire contained all areas recommended for assessment in the music therapy literature with adults, adolescents, and children. In addition, the CTDs were requested to write in any additional areas they assessed that were not listed. From these assessment areas, CTDs were asked to list the five areas they assessed and treated most frequently, and that they felt were most important in music therapy assessment and treatment. CTDs were next requested to list, for each of the five assessment areas they had just listed, two specific problem (nonmusic) behaviors they assess and treat most often. Next to each problem behavior, they also were requested to list two specific music conditions they used to assess and/or treat the problem. The resulting information from this part of the survey was used to construct Part II of the PMTQ, entitled Multimodal Problem Analysis The procedure for obtaining data relating to music assessment was the same as above with the exception that music areas were included. This information was used to construct Part I: Music.

4. Content for Part III: Post Interview Observations was derived from areas clinical training directors assess most frequently during activity therapy assessment. Following is the survey procedure: Areas assessed most frequently during activity therapy assessment were determined by listing in the questionnaire all areas of activity therapy assessment suggested in the music therapy literature. CTDs were requested to choose 10 of the 42 areas listed, then rank order the 10 areas by assigning a 1 to the area they assessed most frequently and a *10* to the area they would assess least frequently. The areas of nonmusic, music, and activity therapy assessment were each listed in alphabetical order, with the order of listing rotated among the questionnaires (CTDs were given a questionnaire for adults, adolescents, or children, depending on the chronological age level which they had previously indicated was their greatest expertise).

5. Patient problems were identified according to the developmental level of the patient, and gender in the case of adults. Developmental level was observed as a function of the degree of illness and chronological age of the patient. Degree of illness was measured by asking CTDs to rate the level of functioning typical of the majority of patients treated in their clinical training program using the Global Assessment of Functioning (GAF) Scale (APA, 1994). Separate questionnaires were designed for adult male and adult female patients.

6. The percentage of CTDs returning the questionnaires for each chronological age level of patient were children, 61%; adolescents, 74%; adult male, 67%; and adult female, 73%.

Descriptive validity. Following the survey analysis, the problems CTDs had indicated they assessed most frequently along with the music therapy interventions, were listed in this manual in the order of frequency in which they were listed by the CTDs. The same procedure was followed for music behavior (See Chapter 1).

Subsequently, the areas and problems assessed in the PMTQ were listed in the same order of frequency in which they were assessed by CTDs, and in which they were listed in this clinical manual. The items in the PMTQ were referenced to the problems in the manual and were written to determine the extent that a patient has the problems. Since the patient population for whom the items were targeted had a mean GAF of 36.5 with a median of 33, the wording of the PMTQ items had to be simplified and could not contain technical terms. For example patient problems such as reclusive, withdrawn behavior was assessed by asking questions such as *I would rather be alone than be with people.*

Following the construction of the PMTQ, it was given to a master's level music therapist and a psychologist who worked with psychiatric patients having the same above GAF scores as the target or survey patient population. The therapists were asked to judge the adequacy of the PMTQ items in terms of (1) whether the items were clear enough so that patients with the above GAF score could understand them, and (2) whether the items assessed the same problems as were listed in this clinical manual (e.g., Did the items lose original meaning in the process of simplification?). Following some minor revisions, both judges independently agreed the PMTQ was sufficient for the purpose for which it was designed.

Functional validity. Popham (1978) defines *functional validity* as the extent that a criterion-referenced test satisfies the purpose to which it is being put. The PMTQ not only provides the music therapist with a profile of the patient's problems, but it also may provide for the establishment of a viable program plan that is satisfactory to the patient and the treatment team. It is suggested however, that the following validity checks be made. After administering the PMTQ the examiner is encouraged to compare the PMTQ results with the results of assessments given by other professionals. The results of the PMTQ frequently are confirmed by other assessments. For example, in the case of *D* described in this chapter, an analysis of *D's* BASIC I.D. indicates poor short and long term memory, persecutory beliefs (Cognitive), hallucinatory perceptions (Sensation), poor leisure skills, and difficulty maintaining long term relationships (Interpersonal) were all independently assessed by D's case history and the PMTQ. The therapist also should check for inconsistencies between the PMTQ and nonmusic therapy assessments. Inconsistencies may be an indication that the patient has not accurately responded to the PMTQ or to other assessments. The examiner should keep in mind however, that the PMTQ is designed to assess problems most frequently treated by music therapists. Nonmusic therapy assessments are not limited to problems assessed most frequently by music therapists and consequently frequently detect patient problems other than those the PMTQ is designed to assess.

Since assessment is an ongoing process, the behavior of the patient in subsequent music therapy sessions also may serve as a measure of the validity of the patient's PMTQ responses. The examiner should note whether the patient's subsequent behavior is consistent or inconsistent with his or her previous PMTQ responses.

It is recommended that additional research also be conducted to supplement the above initial validation of the PMTQ, and that any further validation efforts be consistent with the goals of individualized criterion-referenced, or behavioral assessment. As a behavioral assessment, the PMTQ appears to have adequate content and functional validity for purposes of assessment, program planning, and the implementation of a viable music therapy program.

PART II

PSYCHIATRIC MUSIC THERAPY ASSESSMENTS AND TREATMENTS EMPLOYED IN AMTA-APPROVED CLINICAL TRAINING FACILITIES

CODES

N = Total number of music therapy interventions submitted.

N^1 = Number of music therapy interventions submitted for males for all assessment areas. % = Percentage of N.

N^2 = Number of music therapy interventions submitted for females. % = Percentage of N.

n = Total number of music therapy interventions submitted for a specific area of assessment. % = Percentage of N.

n^1 = Number of music therapy interventions submitted for males within a specific area of assessment. % = Percentage of n.

n^2 = Number of music therapy interventions submitted for females within a specific area of assessment. % = Percentage of n.

n^3 = Number of music therapy interventions submitted for males for a specific problem. % = Percentage of n^5.

n^4 = Number of music therapy interventions submitted for females for a specific problem. % = Percentage of n^5.

n^5 = Total number of music therapy interventions submitted for the specific problem. % = Percentage of n.

—–··—– = Separates different types of music therapy interventions (e.g., playing instruments, singing, composing, moving to music, specified behavior modification techniques, other).

The number(s) after each intervention (e.g., 36) refers to the mean *Global Assessment of Functioning (GAF) Scale* score of patients for whom the intervention was designed. One score was given by each music therapist specifying the intervention (e.g., "25-30-36" indicates the specific intervention was submitted by three music therapists, and that the intervention is used with patients having the above mean GAF scores). See Chapter 1 for a discussion of the GAF Scale.

CHAPTER 3

ADULTS

(Combined, N = 541; Male, N^1 = 260; 48.06% Female, N^2 = 281; 51.94%)

ASSESSMENT AREA – BEHAVIOR
(Combined, n = 55; 10.17%; Male, n^1 = 24; 43.64%; Female, n^2 = 31; 56.36%)

PROBLEM

B-1 Lack of assertiveness resulting in the inability to meet or communicate needs; passivity; difficulty verbalizing needs, feelings, likes and dislikes; does not express own views on a topic during a discussion (n^3 = 5; n^4 = 9; n^5 = 14; 25.45%)

MUSIC THERAPY INTERVENTION

Give patient experience at identifying assertive/nonassertive messages in song lyrics during music listening-discussion activity. M-30; F-30

The patients each select a song to be played during the session. They then work with a partner to negotiate which of the two songs selected will be played for the group. Only one song may be played. M-41; F-41

Encourage controlled, honest verbalization of thoughts, feelings, and needs through the use of certain songs that appeal to the emotions. F-35

The patients each select one song from song books for the group to sing, then tell why they selected the song. M-41; F-41

Have the group sing the song, "My Favorite Things." Each patient will then list the things they enjoy the most and communicate them to the group. M-35; F-32

Have the patient write a song titled "Everybody's Bill of Rights." Let the patient fill in key words. M-51; F-51

Write the lyrics of a familiar song on pieces of cardboard (one lyric written on each piece of cardboard). Seat the group in a circle and distribute the pieces of cardboard to the group members. Ask the group to work together by taking turns finding the words of the song title, or putting the lyrics in order. To achieve this task, each patient must take turns communicating her need for a lyric that a person is holding. F-30

Have the patients toss a ball to one another in the presence of background music. When the music stops, the person holding the ball will verbally respond to a question posed by the therapist. F-30

During the music therapy discussion, call on specific patients, asking each patient to verbalize at least one statement. F-35

B-2 Lack of attention span; does not remain on task long enough to express self; has difficulty concentrating ($n^3 = 4$; $n^4 = 6$; $n^5 = 10$; 18.16%)

Involve patient in structured improvisation over a chordal background. Allow patient to play several instruments during a single session. M-40; F-50

Structure instrumental instruction to enhance on-task behavior and concentration (e.g., plays entire piano composition without stopping). M-51; F-51

Using an alphabet chart (Schulberg, 1981), have the patient rewrite (convert) their name into musical notes. The patient then plays their name on the xylophone followed by improvisation of how they feel or their present mood. F-39

Involve the patient in a hand bell choir in which the patient must ring her assigned bell when the conductor points to her letter on the hand bell chart. F-50

———•—•———

Direct the patient's attention to the musical task (e.g., singing selected song) with verbal reinforcement for completion of the task. M-32; F-39

———•—•———

Involve the patient in a "fill in the blank" song writing activity. M-40; F-50

B-3 Lacks awareness of personal space/boundaries; interrupts others during group discussion; displays inappropriate verbal/nonverbal social behavior toward peers; exhibits lack of boundaries with peers and staff ($n^3 = 4$; $n^4 = 3$; $n^5 = 7$; 12.73%)

Place the resident in a structured music therapy group (e.g., a performing group such as a choir) and provide counseling about proper social skills in group situations; explain the structure and rules of the activity M-25-30; F-31

Conduct one-to-one music therapy sessions with the patient, utilizing activities such as improvisation and musical role playing. M-25

———•—•———

Utilize music and movement activities with an emphasis on space, touch, and boundaries. F-35

———•—•———

Have a group song writing activity which focuses on personal relationships. F-60

———•—•———

During music discussion group, redirect speaking to appropriate times. M-32

B-4 Poor eye contact; difficulty initiating conversation ($n^3 = 3$; $n^4 = 2$; $n^5 = 5$; 9.09%)

Pass a ball around the circle to background music. When the music stops, the patient holding the ball must draw a question from the "hat," read the question, then ask his neighbor the question. M-30

Use a mirroring activity to music. Have the patient select a partner and mirror the partner's movements to increase eye contact and level of comfort. F-60

———

Involve patient in an Orff instrumental activity which requires eye contact for the following of cues. M-30; F-30

———

Require more and more eye contact from the patient. Start by requiring the patient to maintain eye contact momentarily when responding to the therapist at the beginning of the music therapy session. M-33

B-5 Demanding and intrusive (overly assertive) with staff (e.g., States that needs must be met immediately) ($n^3 = 0$; $n^4 = 3$; $n^5 = 3$; 5.45%)

During the music therapy session, have a discussion of personal boundaries and social appropriateness. For example, during music listening-discussion, elicit patient feedback on appropriate ways to confront peers. F-35; F-60

———

During music therapy, have the patients discuss and role play appropriate and reasonable ways to make requests. F-35

B-6 Uses passive dependent, passive aggressive, or aggressive methods of communication rather than being appropriately assertive ($n^3 = 0$; $n^4 = 3$; $n^5 = 3$; 5.45%)

Play the game, Question Ball. The patients pass a ball to recorded or live background music. When the music stops the patient selects a question, reads it aloud, then answers the question. F-30

———

During song writing, have the patients decide on the topic to be reflected by the title, then the title of the song. When composing the song, ask each patient to contribute one or two lines of lyrics/music to the song. F-30

———

Employ assertiveness training techniques combined with various music activities and tasks. F-15

B-7 Lacks self-control; loses temper which may result in tantrums, violence, or arguments with other residents; low frustration tolerance; easily agitated when schedule is disrupted ($n^3 = 2$; $n^4 = 1$; $n^5 = 3$; 5.45%)

Involve the patient in progressive muscle relaxation to music. M-30-25

Use relaxation exercises involving deep breathing while listening to music. F-35

B-8 Exhibits assaultive behavior ($n^3 = 1$; $n^4 = 1$; $n^5 = 3$; 5.45%)

Have the patient freely express anger through the playing of music instruments. Follow by having the patient discuss verbally the reasons for the anger and appropriate solutions. The goal is to get the patient to experience and acknowledge the gratification from using socially acceptable ways to express feelings. M-30; F-30

B-9 Development and channeling of creativity ($n^3 = 1$; $n^4 = 1$; $n^5 = 2$; 3.64%)

Involve patient in music expression activities using Orff techniques. M-30; F-30

B-10 Exhibits rocking behavior while seated ($n^3 = 1$; $n^4 = 1$; $n^5 = 2$; 3.64%)

Conduct standing exercises to music. M-21; F-21

B-11 Complaining behavior ($n^3 = 1$; $n^4 = 1$; $n^5 = 2$; 3.64%)

Utilize a music listening activity in which the patient chooses his favorite music for listening. Follow with a discussion of what the patient likes about the music. Ignore complaints and reinforce noncomplaints. M-21; F-21

B-12 Exhibits general perseverative behaviors ($n^3 = 1$; $n^4 = 0$; $n^5 = 1$; 1.82%)

Utilize success-assured performance tasks such as autoharp strumming. M-30

B-13 Exhibits restless behavior; may have akathisia ($n^3 = 1$; $n^4 = 0$; $n^5 = 1$; 1.82%)

Utilize music and movement activities such as structured dancing. M-30

B-14 Patient, age 50, complains about being in a session with younger patients in their early twenties ($n^3 = 1$; $n^4 = 0$; $n^5 = 1$; 1.82%)

Encourage the older patient to choose music to play for the group, then explain to the group why they like the music. Encourage positive interactions among the patients. M-31

AFFECT
(Combined, n = 121; 22.37%; Male, n^1 = 60; 49.59%; Female, n^2 = 61; 50.41%)

PROBLEM

A-1 Experiences difficulty, or the inability to verbally or nonverbally express/identify feelings/emotions in self or others (e.g., anger, happiness, sadness); difficulty understanding what the other person's feelings may be; restricted emotional expression; lack of congruity between affect and verbalization (e.g., facial expression, vocal tone and volume doesn't match speech content); may exhibit flat affect; emotional detachment; rarely smiles; may acknowledge own inability to experience feelings (n^3 = 28; n^4 = 32; n^5 = 60; 49.59%)

MUSIC THERAPY INTERVENTION

Involve the patient in a song discussion activity, focusing on the affective quality of the song (e.g., Ask the patient: "Is this a happy, sad, angry, or fearful song?) Use songs about specific emotions, such as fear, to help the patient identify and express specific feelings and appropriate ways of expressing them. Prompt generalization to patient's life situation. The overall goal is for the patient to understand and accept feelings as a part of life. M-30-15-25-32-30-30; F-65-41-36-30-15-37-35-31-26

Use music listening, pictures, and imagery to assist the patient in identifying specific feelings elicited by the music. Ask the patient to write any thoughts, feelings, or ideas that emerge while listening to music. Follow with a group discussion of written material. M-15-35; F-15

Have the patient bring songs to the session that express specific feelings related to issues the patient is dealing with during hospitalization. Discuss feelings connected to the songs. M-41; F-41

Ask the patients to pick a song which describes how they feel today. Attempt to elicit the feeling by playing the song. Encourage the patients to "act their feelings" (express their feelings) when talking with the group members. If expression of feeling is not forthcoming, ask the patients to draw their feelings while listening to the song. F-65-31

Encourage patients to verbalize their feelings about songs after they are played, or to identify the feelings of the composer. Use this discussion as a catalyst for focusing on the feelings patients have about their problems. M-25; F-39

Provide the patients with a list of mood states from the Hevner Mood Wheel. Have the patients listen to music, then select the specific mood that best matches the music. F-32

Use high intensity music for listening, followed by a discussion of feeling in the music. Later associate the feeling in the music to bodily sensation, and then to actual feelings within the patient which are representative of the feelings in the music. F-35

Perform different songs with an emotional theme, label the emotion, then discuss situations in the hospital where patients might feel the same. M-26

Ask the patient to bring a song to the group, share the music with the group, then discuss/verbalize her feelings and memories associated with the song, and reasons for sharing the song. F-39

During free or structured improvisation, prompt the patient to identify feelings elicited by the improvisation. The patient may be provided with a checklist of possible feelings to assist in the identification of own feelings. M-30-32; F-30-35-39

From a list of emotions (a "feelings list"), have the patient express musically, with various instruments, each emotion on the list to achieve catharsis. M-51; F-51

Ask the patient to select an emotion from a deck of index cards, each with the name of an emotion. The patient first expresses the emotion using a musical instrument, and then verbally. M-35; F-32

Ask the patient to choose an instrument or instruments from many (i.e., piano, tone bells, Orff xylophone, or other instruments). Have the patient express how she feels by playing the instrument(s). Follow by discussing the feelings with the patient. F-56-35

Have a patient play an emotion on an instrument while the other group members, given visual and aural cues, guess what the emotion is. M-25

Have the patient play and draw their feelings. Follow with a discussion of possible nonmusical outlets for expressing feelings. F-39

During rhythmic improvisation, ask the patient to play her present feelings on an instrument of her choice. The group is then asked if they can identify the patient's feelings. Finally, the patient is asked to verbally describe her feeling to the group. F-60

Ask the patient to choose a song (may be from a list of songs or a song book) that expresses his own feelings or describes himself to the group. The group will then sing and discuss the song. M-33-35-26; F-26-30

Sing songs such as "If You're Happy and You Know It." Follow with role playing of happy, funny, or sad situations/times. M-21; F-21

Utilize voice lessons to develop expression of feelings. M-30; F-60

Involve the patient in a choir in which the patient chooses songs that convey feelings associated with happiness, sadness, death, and relationships. Have the choir sing and discuss such feelings. F-20

Utilize song writing (e.g., The patient portrays an emotion with an instrument such as a drum; the patient expresses own emotions or feelings) M-25-30-60

Utilize a "Blues" writing activity. Patients write "feeling" phrases that may be sung with guitar accompaniment to a 12-bar blues pattern (e.g., "When I'm feelin' _____, I _____.") M-30

_____·_____

Elicit patient participation in music activity of patient's choice while attempting to build a more trusting relationship with the patient. M-45

Present the patient with a box containing labels describing positive emotions. Ask the patient to draw a label from the box, then tell about the time he experienced the emotion described on the label. This technique is useful with patients who experience difficulty talking about past positive life events. M-33

_____·_____

The patient chooses a song that describes his/her feelings. While the song is played, the patient uses the group members to construct (nonverbally) a tableau (sculpture) which shows how he/she is feeling. The patient then explains the tableau. M-35; F-65

A-2 Difficulty or the inability to identify or express emotions regarding a particular life situation; exhibits emotional detachment from life situations (e.g., denies being angry or having worries) ($n^3 = 3$; $n^4 = 5$; $n^5 = 8$; 6.61%)

Use lyric listening to selected music and guided imagery techniques to give the patient experience at associating and recognizing the emotions which accompany life experience. M-30-30; F-41-36-31

Have the patient choose a song which relates to one problem area in her life. F-50

_____·_____

Adapt a song writing activity to facilitate the identification and expression of emotions associated with the life situation. M-51; F-51

A-3 Patient becomes angry when coping with frustration; has difficulty coping with frustration or controlling resulting anger; experiences anger, stress, and frustration which may result in impulsive behavior; verbally hostile when frustrated ($n^3 = 6$; $n^4 = 2$; $n^5 = 8$; 6.61%)

Ask the patient to select, from a listing of song titles that express frustration, a title that best describes his own feelings. M-35-30; F-32

Implement relaxation techniques to diffuse anger. M-75

_____·_____

Teach the patient a new musical skill. Give the patient experience at breaking down musical tasks into small steps which are more easily attainable. Facilitate patient's generalization of this organizational principle (breaking down tasks) to the patient's life situation. M-30-40; F-30

Encourage the patient to channel feelings into more constructive outlets, such as participating in a music activity (e.g., a performing group). M-75

Utilize a variety of techniques: listen to song lyrics about anger; have the patient draw a picture of anger; ask the patient to write a list of anything/anyone who makes him angry; encourage the patient to discuss anger with the group, share coping strategies, and receive feedback (e.g., new ways to cope with anger). M-35

A-4 Hyperactivity; exhibits excitability behaviors; excessive energy levels; agitation; manic behavior (e.g., excessive talking, waving arms) during manic stage ($n^3 = 4$; $n^4 = 2$; $n^5 = 6$; 4.96%)

Utilize group singing with song sheets to elicit behavior which is incompatible with excitatory behavior. M-21; F-21

Utilize singing or singing during structured dances to channel energy. Use patient-preferred music of medium tempo with many lyrics. M-40

Utilize the isorhythmic principle; vector toward relaxing music. M-45-30; F-60

A-5 Depression associated with decreased energy level; has difficulty engaging in tasks because of depression/anhedonia; may recall only sad experiences; expresses hopelessness; pessimistic about future ($n^3 = 3$; $n^4 = 3$; $n^5 = 6$; 4.96%)

Involve the patient in a small group (not all depressed patients) music listening-discussion session. Use music that is of a moderate tempo (not too slow or "upbeat"), and encourage patients to share their musical interests and experiences. M-40; F-50

Utilize success-assured tasks such as the patient selecting records to share with others, or asking the patient to choose a song he likes. M-30

Have the patient choose a song that describes how she feels, and one describing how she would like to feel (e.g., the patient expresses a hopeless, pessimistic feeling, but would like to feel more optimistic about her future). Discuss thoughts, actions, and other factors that may result in feeling more optimistic. F-30

Provide positive experiences through individual or group singing. F-50

Ask the patient to choose a song that she sang when she was young. After singing the song, ask the patient to "share with the group" (tell about) a special childhood friend. F-50

Utilizing a variable speed record player, involve the patient in simple stretching to music, followed by simple movement to a faster tempo. Use a song such as "Lake Song" from the motion picture, *On Golden Pond.* M-26

A-6 Severe depression accompanied by fear of real and imagined events; exhibits sad affect and states a desire to die; suicidal ideation; depressed affect; may exhibit loud, wild, screaming and crying ($n^3 = 4$; $n^4 = 2$; $n^5 = 6$; 4.96%)

Ask the patient to listen to music (recorded or live) and to experience the feelings she believes to be overwhelming. Utilize the group for support, and in the discussion of survival and coping strategies. F-39

Elicit positive statements or gestures from patient during selected music listening activity. M-30

Listen to and discuss the song, "Don't Give Up." Help patient relate to present life situation (e.g., severe depression; suicidal ideation) M-35

———•◦•———

Involve the patient in the singing of familiar songs with a focus on validating own current emotions. F-25

———•◦•———

Provide the patient with positive experiences at group instrumental performance or group singing. M-40

———•◦•———

Involve the group in the playing of musical games to elicit positive group affect (the goal is to get the depressed patient to also experience the positive affect). F-25

———•◦•———

Assist patient in developing the ability to concentrate on musical involvement to the exclusion, at least temporarily, of disturbing thoughts. M-40

A-7 Free floating anxiety; not relaxed; easily frustrated; reports high level of anxiety about life situation; inability to relax; may be evidenced by muscle rigidity, sleep disturbance, verbal fretting, or verbal rumination ($n^3 = 3$; $n^4 = 1$; $n^5 = 4$; 3.31%)

Utilize relaxation with music. Encourage the patient to relax while listening. M-25

Schedule the patient for water relaxation whereby floatation and music are combined. M-75

Teach appropriate relaxation procedures which patients can use outside of treatment groups. M-39

———•◦•———

Incorporate breathing and muscle relaxation exercises into vocal music instruction. Present progressively slower tempos to aid body-mind relaxation. F-35

A-8 Impulsive emotional outbursts such as inappropriate laughing, crying, or anger; behavior may become unmanageable during periods of frustration; lacks self-control or impulse control ($n^3 = 3$; $n^4 = 1$; $n^5 = 4$; 3.31%)

Involve the patient in a structured rhythm stick activity to rhythmic, stimulative music (e.g., Use the song, "Beat It."). M-30; F-30

Choose musical conditions which serve as outlets for the expression of more socially acceptable behavior. Channel the energy into a music activity and control for inappropriate behavior. M-45; F-26

Involve the patient in progressive muscle relaxation to music. F-30

Ask the patient if the response is related to the musical experience; direct the patient to the musical task. M-32

A-9 Panic attacks ($n^3 = 2$; $n^4 = 2$; $n^5 = 4$; 3.31%)

Music is utilized in a listening and/or imagery experience to aid in helping the patient to learn relaxation techniques. M-41; F-41

Instill a conditioned relaxation response to aid management of panic attacks. M-51; F-51

A-10 Angry emotional outbursts often resulting in violence; may be diagnosed as Intermittent Explosive Disorder; short temper tantrums sometimes resulting in violence; difficulty responding to verbal feedback without becoming explosive/hostile towards self or others ($n^3 = 0$; $n^4 = 3$; $n^5 = 3$; 2.48%)

During the music therapy session, encourage the patient to express intense feelings while maintaining control. F-35

Play Phil Collins's "I Don't Care Anymore." Discuss the patient's anger. Have the patient write two lists, one listing ways the patient presently copes with anger, and the other listing healthier ways to deal with anger. F-65

Redirect the behavior before it escalates (e.g., offer to let the patient listen to music through the Walkman; conduct music relaxation activities). F-25

A-11 Patient feels emotionally "out of control" when listening to certain songs ($n^3 = 1$; $n^4 = 1$; $n^5 = 2$; 1.65%)

Songs evoking "scary" or "out of control" feelings should be explored with the therapist. Discuss and explore songs, feelings, and issues related to the songs. M-41; F-41

A-12 Difficulty identifying and expressing own feelings which are perceived as being unacceptable (i.e., anger or fear); inability or difficulty recognizing suppressed feelings ($n^3 = 2$; $n^4 = 0$; $n^5 = 2$; 1.65%)

Song discussions using carefully selected music which represents the patient's latent emotions. Observe for identification and projection. M-40

Use referential improvisations on poignant subjects with subsequent discussion. M-40

A-13 Patient experiences anger when the focus of attention is on other patients ($n^3 = 0$; $n^4 = 1$; $n^5 = 1$; 00.83%)

Sing and discuss songs about sharing and noticing the needs of others. M-33

A-14 Displays affect which is inappropriate to the situation ($n^3 = 1$; $n^4 = 0$; $n^5 = 1$; 00.83%)

Have the patient improvise a sound pattern then verbalize the expressed emotion. F-32

A-15 Intellectualizes feelings ($n^3 = 0$; $n^4 = 1$; $n^5 = 1$; 00.83%)

During lyric analysis, after listening to a selection, ask the patient to identify the feelings expressed in the lyrics. Next ask the patient to associate these feelings with similar feelings she is experiencing in the present, or has experienced in the past. F-60

A-16 Inability or unwillingness to empathize with others ($n^3 = 1$; $n^4 = 0$; $n^5 = 1$; 00.83%)

A patient selects a three by five inch card from a set of "emotion cards," then improvises the emotion indicated on the card. Another patient is asked to attempt to identify the emotion from the improvisation, and explain why the first patient chose the particular emotion. M-40

A-17 Alternates between manic and depressive episodes; exhibits behavioral extremes ($n^3 = 0$; $n^4 = 1$; $n^5 = 1$; 00.83%)

Redirect by involving the patient in expressive music activities such as song writing and improvisation. Use sedative or stimulative music. F-37

A-18 Difficulty relating to staff that is the same sex as the abuser (e.g., female resents male staff) ($n^3 = 0$; $n^4 = 1$; $n^5 = 1$; 00.83%)

Provide individual music lessons from a therapist who is the same sex as the abuser. Gradually explore the patient's feelings as an alliance is established. F-31

A-19 Patient feels severe rage at mother for not providing protection during times of abuse ($n^3 = 0$; $n^4 = 1$; $n^5 = 1$; 00.83%)

Involve the patient in a choir led by a female music therapist to give the patient experience at working with a female authority figure. F-31

SENSORY
(Combined, n = 20; 3.70%; Male, n^1 = 10; 50.00%; Female, n^2 = 10; 50.00%)

PROBLEM

S-1 Patient is preoccupied with internal thoughts; hallucinates; auditory hallucinations (e.g., hears voices); talks to ones self ($n^3 = 3$; $n^4 = 6$; $n^5 = 9$; 45.00%)

MUSIC THERAPY INTERVENTION

Play patient-preferred music during a listening-discussion activity. Redirect the patient's attention from internal events to interacting in group discussion about the music. Suggested discussion topics may focus on the music content, or patient ratings of the song. M-40; F-30

During listening-discussion group give the patient experience at focusing on and distinguishing between internal and external stimuli. F-35

———•+•———

Encourage on-task behavior in a music group (e.g., singing). M-25; F-26

Have the patient follow song lyrics by singing, reading, or listening to music in a small group. F-30

———•+•———

Utilize concrete, task-oriented activities (e.g., playing, strumming, or pushing chords on the autoharp, or playing/improvising on other instruments) to assist the patient in focusing on one task at a time. M-30; F-60-32

S-2 Patient experiences difficulty coping with stress and tension; may result in insomnia, withdrawal, chaotic behavior, aggression, isolating self; refusing medications, substance abuse and/or other inappropriate behavior ($n^3 = 7$; $n^4 = 4$; $n^5 = 11$; 55.00%)

Combine music with progressive relaxation techniques and guided imagery. Follow with a discussion of stress and methods of coping. M-15-30-30; F-39-30-15

Encourage the patient to attend a relaxation group which focuses on progressive muscle relaxation and breathing exercises. Follow with a statement from the patient as to the level of relaxation achieved. M-75

Teach progressive muscle relaxation using music to elicit the responses. M-30

Use music listening combined with muscle relaxation. Use music agreed upon by the patient and the therapists. M-40

Use lyric discussions to help facilitate problem solving of adequate, successful coping skills. M-15; F-15

IMAGERY
(Combined, n = 2; 00.37%; Male, n^1 = 2; 100.00%; Female, n^2 = 0; 00.00%)

PROBLEM

IM-1 Difficulty envisioning a pleasant place during progressive relaxation (n^3 = 1; n^4 = 0; n^5 = 1; 50.00%)

MUSIC THERAPY INTERVENTION

Have the patient get comfortably situated then play background music. Ask the patient, "What do you picture when listening to this music selection?" M-30

IM-2 Difficulty focusing on pleasant place for 10–15 minutes (n^3 = 1; n^4 = 0; n^5 = 1; 50.00%)

Have the patient watch a videotape of his attempted relaxation. Analyze the tape for any aural and/or visual clues as to why the patient is having difficulty. M-30

IM-3 Distorted body image (associated with eating disorder) (n^3 = 0; n^4 = 1; n^5 = 30; 50.00%)

Use music with progressive muscle relaxation to help the patient develop body awareness, or a realistic body image. F-31

COGNITIVE
(Combined, n = 112; 20.70%; Male, n^1 = 45; 40.18%; Female, n^2 = 67; 59.82%)

PROBLEM

C-1 Low self-esteem; reports feelings of worthlessness; expresses low opinion of self; makes negative self-statements; exhibits problems talking to others because of low self-esteem; has difficulty expressing positive aspects about self; lacks the necessary self-confidence to try to overcome life problems or to try new activities; convinced they are destined for failure; may feel they have no special skills, or that they can't do anything meaningful; discounts compliments (n^3 = 10; n^4 = 20; n^5 = 30; 26.79%)

MUSIC THERAPY INTERVENTION

Utilize instrumental or vocal music therapy activities to produce a positive experience either individually or in a group. Utilize success oriented music activities to enhance self-esteem (e.g., playing the Omnichord; encourage instrumental experimentation and improvisation). Engineer the instrumental performance to produce patient feelings of success, accomplishment, and peer acceptance. M-30-51-25-25; F-30-51-39-39-60

Teach the patient to play a musical instrument (e.g., guitar or piano) or give voice lessons (depending upon capabilities). During lessons, have the patient point out at least one positive aspect of their playing. M-35-30; F-41-32-65-60

——•·•——

Involve patient in lyric analysis-discussion activities. M-40; F-50-39

Have patients listen to and choose songs about positive self-statements. As a follow-up, have each patient construct a list of positive self-statements to keep with them, and to review when they start thinking negative statements about themselves (e.g., Use the song, "Desiderata" to explore positive aspects of self). M-26; F-26-39

Play Billy Joel's, "Just the Way You Are." Discuss the idea of accepting yourself as you are. Ask each patient to "List on a piece of paper, three things you like about yourself." Have the patients pass their papers around the group so each group member can add something else they like about each patient. F-65

Have the patient choose a song title that represents her. F-28

——•·•——

Involve the patient in song composition activities. M-35; F-50

Arrange for the patient to learn a new skill such as song writing. M-40

——•·•——

Have the patient draw to selected music. Follow with interpretation and discussion. F-41-50

——•·•——

Play musical games which require paired teams such as "Music Pictionary." F-50

Have the patient make an album cover that represents her. F-28

C-2 Delusions; expresses delusional ideas; paranoid ideation (e.g., patient accuses the therapist of saying things against the patient); has difficulty accepting reality; may perceive actions of others as potential threats; excessively concerned with protecting one's own interest; does not trust peers ($n^3 = 5$; $n^4 = 9$; $n^5 = 14$; 12.50%)

Redirect discussion to reality oriented statements (e.g., ask the patient identify the names of instruments or the performer in a music recording) M-30; F-32

Play a song about concrete concepts (e.g., "This Land Is Your Land"). During the discussion probe for reality statements from the patient (e.g., Where were you born? When were you born? What is your present address?). M-26; F-26

Utilize a music listening-discussion session in which the patient is encouraged to sit with the other group members. Encourage the patient to talk about and choose music that makes them feel more comfortable towards others. F-20

Involve the patient in a lyric discussion group with the eventual goal of the patient sharing her own music with the group. F-39

During music-listening, arrange for the patient to get group feedback concerning ideas in a song which are similar to ideas in the patient's delusions. M-25

Discuss why certain topics of discussion for social situations and settings are appropriate or inappropriate. Involve the patient in various social uses of music, such as background music for discussion and dancing. F-30

Involve patient in activities such as social mirroring dances and musical charades. M-35

Arrange for the patient to experience trust. Using a recording of the song, "Lean on Me," have the patients form a circle, hold hands, then lean back so that the group supports each other's weight. F-30

Sing songs with lyrics that reinforce positive self-esteem. M-35; F-30

Redirect the patient's focus to concentrating on a musical project. Getting the patient involved in playing an instrument, if interested, is especially effective at redirecting delusional conversation. F-37

During music therapy session do activities which require sharing and trusting. F-37

C-3 Lacks problem-solving skills; inability to view alternatives to problems; inappropriate coping mechanisms (drinking, drug abuse, verbal/physical aggression; feeling overwhelmed); difficulty organizing tasks; difficulty identifying logical steps toward accomplishing a goal; may view problems as being unmanageable; lacks insight; has difficulty managing problems occurring both on the hospital unit and outside the hospital ($n^3 = 4$; $n^4 = 9$; $n^5 = 13$; 11.61%)

Involve the patient in lyric analysis and song writing activities. Prompt the patient to find solutions to problems reflected in the song lyrics, the patients life, or both. Employ role reversal techniques. M-40; F-50-26-28

After singing the song, "Gonna Lay Down My Burdens," have the patients identify a burden (problem) they are experiencing, and at least one step they can take toward a resolution. Rewrite into the song all the information gained about burdens and their resolutions. F-39

Utilizing Blues form, write a Blues song allowing patients to vent in the first verse, their frustrations over unsolved problems. Follow with a discussion about how to solve the problems and cope with the frustration. Write the resulting solutions and coping mechanisms into the second verse of the song. F-39

Cut each staff line from a piece of sheet music (complete song). Mix up the pieces of paper, each containing a staff line, then ask the patient to reassemble or reconstruct the music so the therapist can use the music to sing the song. F-56

Using a song such as "Bridge over Troubled Waters," have the group identify problems they have experienced, and various ways they have coped with the problems. F-39

During music listening-discussion, have the patient identify both appropriate and inappropriate coping skills heard in songs. M-40

Select the song, "Logical Song" by Super Tramp for listening-discussion. Ask the patients to identify a goal and draw a road map which shows how they will achieve the goal. F-56

Play Twila Paris's, "The Warrior Is a Child." Have the patients draw a personal shield. On the shield, have the patients draw/list things they have in their life that help to provide them with motivation. F-65

Implement stress management and relaxation techniques. M-35

Observe the patient's ability to obey rules during group improvisation (e.g., "Only one person can play at a time."). M-40

C-4 Disorientation; difficulty with orientation (person, place, and time), memory/attention span; lacks reality orientation; loose associations; may be caused by physical illness such as Organic Brain Syndrome or Alzheimer's disease ($n^3 = 5$; $n^4 = 7$; $n^5 = 12$; 10.71%)

Utilize song discussion (after singing or listening to a familiar song) to encourage the patient to express specific reality oriented statements (e.g., about past or present events). Redirect inappropriate responses. M-41-32-30; F-41-60

———•—

Utilize musical games such as Name That Tune, or filling in the blank (missing lyric) on song sheets. F-31-30

Play the game, Question Ball. The patients pass a ball to recorded or live background music. When the music stops the patient selects a question, reads it aloud, then answers the question (This activity may need to be adapted to the functioning level of the patient.). F-30

———•—

Complete a questionnaire on the patient's musical preferences (part of the music therapy assessment). Perform a simple arrangement of a popular song (e.g., "The Rose") on the metallophones. Ask the patient to play a "C" and say his name, or play a "G" and say his neighbor's name. M-26

Involve the patient in an activity that requires reality oriented behavior, such as playing instruments in rhythm and with correct chords. Elicit appropriate comments and maintain on-task behavior. F-41

———•—

Involve the patient in a very structured activity, such as drawing to music. M-35

C-5 Exhibits poor short/long term memory skills; difficulty remembering names ($n^3 = 2$; $n^4 = 3$; $n^5 = 5$; 4.46%)

Ask the patient to identify their music preferences during a sing-a-long activity. Follow by performing the preferred songs. F-32

After the patient finishes singing a song, ask the patient to recall the name of the song. M-30

Have the patient recall music patterns, such as the rhythm or the melody, during the session. M-32

———•—

Practice short-term recall by asking the patient questions about the song lyrics. F-41

———•—

Ask the patient to name each instrument used in a given improvisation session. F-25

C-6 Poor decision-making skills; may have difficulty making daily life decisions or recognizing own erroneous decisions ($n^3 = 2$; $n^4 = 3$; $n^5 = 5$; 4.46%)

During the music therapy session have the patient select from among two or more instruments which instrument he will play. M-32

Ask the patient to orchestrate and lead a small group improvisation based on a selected title card (e.g., "Rain Storm"). M-40

Given a list of songs ask the patient to choose one song for group singing. Also, given two favorite songs, the patient must choose one for group singing. F-31

Given a tape recording containing various songs, have the patient select one song for listening and discussion. The lyrics of the song must describe a coping skill. F-60

Have the patient choose from a variety of activities such as instrumental, vocal, or listening, and from materials associated with such activities (e.g., tapes, songs, instruments). F-35

C-7 Patient denies having problems; withdraws from problems; exhibits resistance to treatment during therapy or hospitalization ($n^3 = 3$; $n^4 = 1$; $n^5 = 4$; 3.57%)

Discuss song lyrics that relate to the patient's problems; choose songs for lyric analysis that focus the patient on specific therapeutic issues. M-30-41; F-30

Provide a relaxed/nonthreatening music experience (e.g., learning the guitar, music listening) to encourage trust and increase personal insight through gentle redirection by the therapist. M-41

C-8 Patient has difficulty accepting responsibility for change; has difficulty accepting change in basic daily routine ($n^3 = 2$; $n^4 = 1$; $n^5 = 3$; 2.68%)

Involve the patient in a success-oriented, very structured music therapy activity (e.g., Orff instrumental activity). Gradually increase patient responsibility and change variables as the patient feels more comfortable with the group. M-35; F-32

Employ structured improvisation (e.g., on the song "La Bamba") followed by the changing of instruments (regardless of the patient's choice of instrument). Follow with a discussion relating to change. M-26

C-9 Gives up easily when solving problems; easily frustrated; inability to cope with failure; goes to bed upon not being successful ($n^3 = 1$; $n^4 = 2$; $n^5 = 3$; 2.68%)

Involve the patient in a dyadic improvisation with the music therapist. The patient selects a three by five card instructing him to, in some manner, change the improvisation of the therapist. Observe frustration threshold. M-40

Teach the patient a music performance skill. Insure a reasonable amount of success, but remind the patient that all persons make mistakes when learning to play a music instrument. Generalize principle to real life situations. F-50

———•+•———

Have a discussion of song lyrics which pertain to the relationship between perseverance and success. F-30

C-10 Difficulty following directions; inability or unwillingness to listen to or comprehend directions ($n^3 = 0$; $n^4 = 3$; $n^5 = 3$; 2.68%)

Demonstrate a music task to the patient (e.g., how to play a tambourine). As the patient's ability to follow directions improves, increase the task complexity (e.g., teach one rhythm pattern, then two rhythm patterns, etc.) F-32

During instrumental improvisation, give the patient simple one or two step directions about how to play a percussion instrument. F-25

———•+•———

Make group rules and directions for music activities exceptionally clear and easy to understand. F-37

C-11 Patient is unaware of the purpose or need for hospitalization; may be resistive to treatment ($n^3 = 1$; $n^4 = 1$; $n^5 = 2$; 1.79%)

Encourage patient discussion of personal needs during reflective song discussion groups. M-35

———•+•———

Provide a relaxed, nonthreatening music experience (e.g., learning guitar, listening) to encourage trust and increase personal insights through gentle redirection by the therapist. F-41

C-12 Patient has difficulty accepting or coping with the reality of hospitalization; may feel hopeless and discouraged ($n^3 = 0$; $n^4 = 2$; $n^5 = 2$; 1.79%)

Have the group members compose a parody to the song, "Please Release Me." F-30

———•+•———

Have the group listen to the song, "There's a Place in the Sun." Follow with a discussion of what gives them encouragement, and how they can find additional sources of encouragement. F-30

C-13 Patient admits own problems, but denies others may have similar problems. ($n^3 = 1$; $n^4 = 1$; $n^5 = 2$; 1.79%)

Involve the patient in a lyric analysis discussion about general life problems and ways to cope with them. M-35; F-32

C-14 Patient experiences difficulties with verbal therapy because of low level of functioning (e.g., chronic disorder) ($n^3 = 1$; $n^4 = 1$; $n^5 = 2$; 1.79%)

Involve the patient in rhythmic activities (e.g., playing rhythm instruments to accompany songs) to elicit physical involvement and organization of thoughts. M-41; F-41

C-15 Delusions of grandeur (e.g., unrealistic aspirations to be a "rock star"); maintains delusional system regarding self as a famous musician ($n^3 = 0$; $n^4 = 2$; $n^5 = 2$; 1.79%)

For unrealistic "rock star' aspirations, involve the patient in reading and discussing biographies of musical performers, especially "rock stars." Follow by assigning musical tasks according to ability. F-37

Use a gradual progression of activities, beginning with involving the patient in playing/singing, then audio taping the patient, and next videotaping the patient. The goal is to confront the patient's delusional system, while fostering a more realistic patient perception of actual skills and abilities. Reinforce and develop the patient's real strengths. F-35

C-16 Demonstrates poor judgment; difficulty assessing social situations and following appropriate protocol ($n^3 = 2$; $n^4 = 0$; $n^5 = 2$; 1.79%)

Following the discussion of a musical style preferred by the group, ask the patient to select, from a variety of styles, music to which the group would like to listen. M-32

Ask the patient to supply the appropriate solution (i.e., "Fill in the blank") to a variety of problematic social situations. M-40

C-17 Lack of self-awareness ($n^3 = 1$; $n^4 = 0$; $n^5 = 1$; 00.89%)

Involve patient in music relaxation and discussion to help patient become more aware of present life situation. M-35

C-18 Difficulty with setting goals ($n^3 = 1$; $n^4 = 0$; $n^5 = 1$; 00.89%)

Involve the patient in a goal sharing group. The patients listen to goal-related songs, then each patient writes a time line for future specific goals. M-30

C-19 Misinterprets messages/communications from others ($n^3 = 0$; $n^4 = 1$; $n^5 = 1$; 00.89%)

Use instruments to role play conversations, arguments, conflicts, or other personal experiences. Discuss patient perceptions of the type of communication that took place during the improvisations (e.g., Angry conversation? Casual conversation? Was the conflict settled?). F-39

C-20 Feelings of helplessness ($n^3 = 1$; $n^4 = 0$; $n^5 = 1$; 00.89%)

Involve the patient in a reflective discussion of song lyrics that relate to the patient's problem. M-35

C-21 Lacks ability to structure time, manage a limited budget, and utilize community resources ($n^3 = 1$; $n^4 = 0$; $n^5 = 1$; 00.89%)

Conduct group singing of songs about efficient community living. Follow with group discussion. M-25

C-22 Difficulty or inability to relate to metaphor ($n^3 = 1$; $n^4 = 0$; $n^5 = 1$; 00.89%)

During song discussion, encourage the patient to explain own interpretation of the lyrical metaphor used in the song. M-40

C-23 Lacks concept of a healthy heterosexual relationship; becomes involved in destructive relationships resulting in emotional and physical abuse ($n^3 = 0$; $n^4 = 1$; $n^5 = 1$; 00.89%)

Conduct lyric discussions of songs having themes related to the patient's problems (e.g., intimacy, loneliness, dependency, friendship, support). F-35

INTERPERSONAL-SOCIALIZATION
(Combined, n = 177; 32.72%; Male, n^1 = 96; 54.24% %; Female, n^2 = 81; 45.76 %)
Includes LEISURE SKILLS

PROBLEM

IS-1 Reclusive; withdrawn; isolative behavior; minimal personal interactions; does not feel comfortable or relate to others when in group; little or no verbalization; may not initiate conversation; may be preoccupied with personal problems or depressed ($n^3 = 28$; $n^4 = 34$; $n^5 = 62$; 35.28%)

MUSIC THERAPY INTERVENTION

Involve the patient in music listening and discussion of the lyrics, artist, or other musical characteristics. Wait for the patient to respond. M-25-30-21-32-31; F-30-21-39

Utilize a record selection activity, where patients are paired off and asked to select a song to which they can both relate. Although the activity goal is to facilitate peer interaction, group discussion may also be facilitated. M-30-25

Involve the group in writing a story about the group which is set to instrumental background music, with the goal of facilitating verbalization and interaction. M-51; F-51

Ask the patient to collaborate with his neighbor in determining five singers whom they both like. M-33; F-30

Tape a piece of paper on each patient's back. Play the song, "That's What Friends Are For," then have each patient write on the back of each patient, one positive quality about the patient. M-35; F-32

After listening to songs such as, "You've Got a Friend," "That's What Friends Are For," and "There's a Winner in You," the patient must state a positive quality about the peer seated on the right, the left, and herself. F-60

Involve the patient in a group music therapy session in which each patient picks a record that describes herself, then tells the group why. F-20

As an exercise in negotiating skills, ask the patients to choose, from a stack of 10 albums, only two songs for listening. M-85

Establish initial participation by presenting a music activity in which the patient is interested. Follow by gradually involving the patient in music listening-discussion of musical selections significant to the patient's problems. M-45

To promote the sharing of music experiences, assign each patient to bring to the session the music of their favorite artist, and give a presentation to the rest of the group. M-80

Choose music for discussion which describes positive qualities possessed by all group members. F-60

Give one-to-one instrumental instruction to establish rapport and trust. Prepare the patient for participation in a music ensemble, or to play a solo, with the goal of increasing interpersonal interaction. F-36-31-31

Play "Stop the Music." The patients pass a rhythm instrument around the group while the music plays. When the music stops, the patient holding the instrument chooses a card from the "grab bag." The patient reads the card to the person on his left, who in turn must answer the question. M-21; F-56-21

Present group improvisation on a variety of instruments, letting patients take turns directing. The director indicates through hand positions what the group is to do (e.g., get louder, higher, or lower). During the following discussion, present questions such as, "What does it feel like to be in front of people, or to be a leader? How did you communicate? Do we ever need to change our communication techniques? F-31-26

Arrange the conditions in a music performance group so patients must listen to other performers in order to match pitches and rhythms. F-37

Conduct structured improvisation without verbal interaction (i.e., begin with having the patient mimic an answer/response). F-35

Select an improvisation activity requiring the patient to choose a partner, or one in which two patients play simultaneously. M-40

Create an improvisation using two xylophones. Instruct two group members to have a "conversation" using only the instruments to "talk." Follow with a discussion of the interaction. F-39

Place the resident in a performing group. Encourage interaction and conversation with other residents. M-25

Ask the patient to choose a group member to trade instruments with, and to name the group member. F-25

Involve the patient in group singing with an emphasis on cooperative interpersonal interaction. M-51-25

During group singing, promote patient recall of the names of group members. Songs which require the greeting or naming of peers may be used. M-30; F-30

Ask the patient to collaborate with her neighbor in choosing a song for the group to sing. F-26

During the music therapy session, have the patient introduce their peers or neighbor and tell something about them. Facilitator songs may be used, such as "Getting to Know You." F-35

During a talent show or sing-a-long arrange conditions for patient interaction (e.g., sharing song books, sharing microphone, singing with peers). F-35

Play the following game: Arrange the group in a circle and have the members throw a ball to whomever they wish while the music plays. When the music stops, the person holding the ball must tell something good about the person who threw the ball. M-21; F-21

Encourage group interaction by involving the patient in musical games (e.g., Pictionary, Musical Bingo). F-28

Facilitate structured interaction through musical games (e.g., Music Trivia, a dice game). F-65

Involve the patient in movement/dance activities. M-35-40

Develop nonverbal interaction skills by having the patient participate in mirroring to music. F-26

Introduce a music and movement task with defined space limitations (i.e., the patient must remain in the circle or square). M-32

During song composition, compose parodies (rewriting the lyrics of familiar songs) to describe each group member (e.g., name, feeling) or on group themes. Sing the parodies during group singing. F-35-30

Utilizing a song writing activity (e.g., fill in the blanks technique), assist the patient in identifying a hierarchy of social activities, perceived by the patient from least to most threatening. Have the patient make one hierarchy for hospital and one for community social activities. M-40

Each patient will write a poem, read the poem aloud to the group, and then orchestrate the poem. Encourage group members to volunteer to play instruments and to assist where needed. F-39

Conduct structured interviews to determine musical interests. Appoint partners with similar interests to share their interests with the group. M-26; F-26

Have the patient design an album cover complete with art work and song titles that describe her. Upon completion, the patient is asked to show the finished album to the group and talk about it. F-56

Arrange for the patients to work on a project together, such as putting together a display featuring various music groups. M-85

Build self-esteem through positive musical experiences. M-30

Encourage the patient to attend a small music variety group (two-four members), and participate in activities such as group singing, rhythm band, and informal "jam" sessions. During the activities, encourage the patient to respond to the therapist's questions. M-75

Use music activities that encourage the patients to make nonintimidating contact with one another (e.g., physical contact, verbal contact, eye contact). F-35

IS-2 Does not utilize leisure time; has difficulty constructively managing or structuring leisure time; indicates a lack of "things to do"; frequently does nothing, sleeps, or watches television; poor leisure skills; lacks leisure skills; no hobbies or interests ($n^3 = 20$; $n^4 = 12$; $n^5 = 32$; 18.08%)

Demonstrate different styles of music to find out the patient's likes and dislikes. Provide 20–30 minutes each day for listening. Reinforce behavior. M-21-30; F-21

Provide leisure education about community activities and music as leisure. Take the patient on field trips to community music events such as concerts and recitals. M-35; F-36-30

Teach the patient to pursue personal music interests, such as providing training on how to buy a stereo and build a tape library. M-30; F-30

Use guided imagery and music to help the patient explore leisure interests. M-26; F-26

Ask patient to express leisure interests/skills by drawing to music. M-26; F-26

Develop healthy ways of structuring free time by taking patients on field trips to community events such as concerts, plays and museums. M-30

Develop music performance skills such as piano or guitar playing for use as leisure after discharge. Have the patient compile a notebook of songs and chords learned. Arrange performance opportunities for the patient. M-30-25-25-26-75-40-30-30; F-60-30-31

Teach the patient a musical skill which can be used in the community (e.g., singing in the church choir). M-30; F-50-26

Have the patient construct a "leisure collage" by looking through magazines and cutting out pictures of leisure activities. Sing related songs such as "My Favorite Things." F-35

Teach music theory to the patient if some music performance abilities are present. M-26

Assist the patient in composing a song, then publish the song in the hospital newsletter. M-40

Start with simple stretching activities to music, then progress to dance (e.g., Country and Western, Rock, Polka). M-31

Prepare the patient for re-entry into the community by explaining community music recreational opportunities. Prepare patient for participation. M-45

IS-3 Uncooperative behavior in group settings; uncooperative with staff and patients; disruptive; breaks rules; interrupts; does not change behavior to conform to rules; chooses to not follow directions ($n^3 = 8$; $n^4 = 9$; $n^5 = 17$; 9.61%)

Involve the patient in a music "combo" activity such as a choir. Cultivate group awareness and cohesion. M-30-40-30-30; F-30

Involve the patient in group singing to enhance cooperative interpersonal interaction. F-51

Using resonator bells or tone chimes, assign a bell to each group member. Emphasize the importance of following directions and working together to achieve the final product. M-35-40; F-35-32

Pair patients into groups of two or more. Ask them to plan, practice, and perform a music selection, with each taking a turn at playing a solo while accompanied by the other members of the instrumental group. F-32

First work with the patient on a one-to-one basis to prepare for integration into a music ensemble. M-30; F-60

Involve the patient in a music activity of choice with as much individual attention as possible. If the uncooperative behavior does not improve, remove the patient from the group for one week. F-37

When planning a music therapy activity, involve the patient in the formulation of "reasonable" rules for the activity. F-37

Ask the patient to work with another patient in assigning a rating (1 through 10) to a selection of music. F-25

Involve the patient in musical team games such as Music Trivia, Music Bingo, and Musical Chairs. M-40

IS-4 Lack of interest and motivation to use leisure time; is not motivated to engage in leisure activities; boredom resulting from a lack of interests; may choose watching television/ smoking as only leisure activities; has limited leisure skills; has few friends ($n^3 = 8$; $n^4 = 5$; $n^5 = 13$; 7.36%)

Improve musical skills to develop interests in music leisure activities. Give the patient the opportunity to discover past skills or to use existing skills. One approach may be to use lyric analysis to discuss types of music skills, with the goal of remotivating the patient to use such skills. M-35-40; F-50

Utilize music listening activities to identify musical interests and to increase motivation to use music as leisure. M-30; F-30

Refer the patient to a listening laboratory in which he can accumulate points for each 20 minutes of music listening. Points can then be exchanged for numerous items (excluding cigarettes). M-21; F-21

Utilize music listening activities to teach the patient about music they may enjoy. Incorporate group discussion to stimulate verbal interaction with peers. M-31

———•·•———

Involve the patient in leisure music activities that would prepare the patient for musical opportunities in her home town, such as square dancing, theatrical groups, or social dances. F-20

Use music passively as background music to nonmusic recreational activities, such as physical exercise, walking, and lifting weights. F-35

———•·•———

Search out musical experiences from past life. If none are found, introduce new ones that are easy to acquire. M-45

Assist patient in discovering musical interests and in developing the use of music as leisure. M-30

———•·•———

Conduct an instrumental improvisation session on the patient's ward. M-25

IS-5 Experiences difficulty in bonding with others as evidenced by lack of friendships and/or excessive marital conflicts; difficulty maintaining long term (more than one year) relationships/friendships; difficulty relating to or feeling comfortable with others ($n^3 = 1$; $n^4 = 4$; $n^5 = 5$; 2.83%)

Utilize group singing to integrate the patient into the "patient community bond." M-15; F-15

———•·•———

Utilize movement games which require interaction with others (e.g., imitation of the movement of others). F-50

———•·•———

During group improvisation, give the patient experience at both leading and following. F-50

———•·•———

Conduct a listening-discussion session of songs that focus on positive aspects of relationships/friendships. Follow by having the patients improvise on instruments the feelings they associate with relationships/friendships. F-35

IS-6 Experiences difficulty with the sharing of personal data, such as likes and dislikes with the group; has difficulty with, or is withdrawn from disclosing personal issues ($n^3 = 2$; $n^4 = 3$; $n^5 = 5$; 2.83%)

After a session in which the patient has disclosed personal issues to the group, sing a bonding song such as "Amazing Grace." M-15; F-15

_____•_•_____

Have the patient bring to the session songs that express specific feelings related to issues the patient is dealing with during hospitalization. Discuss the feelings. F-41

_____•_•_____

During rhythmic improvisation the patient selects a peer group member with whom she needs to share information (e.g., personal issue; problem; concern), but is unable to do so verbally. The patient then shares and exchanges information nonverbally with the peer, each using instrumental improvisation. After the improvisation the patient discusses the information with the peer. F-60

_____•_•_____

Use musical games to help make information sharing nonthreatening to the patient. M-15

IS-7 Has difficulty involving self in community groups; unable to make acquaintances in church or community ($n^3 = 3$; $n^4 = 1$; $n^5 = 4$; 2.26%)

Teach the patient the expectations of a community choir, and develop vocal performance skills. M-30; F-30

Prepare the patient to join a church choir by giving voice lessons and self-confidence training. M-33

Conduct group singing and discussion of songs about friendship and positive relationships. M-25

IS-8 Does not sit with group; sits near the periphery of the group; sits behind group members or alone; continually leaves the room, or stands and watches the group from afar ($n^3 = 3$; $n^4 = 1$; $n^5 = 4$; 2.26%)

Use rhythmic improvisation. Encourage the patient to select an instrument and to participate in ensemble playing with group members. Although the patient may initially remain seated near the periphery of the group while playing, as the patient feels more comfortable, encourage her to assume a more central seating position in the group. F-60

_____•_•_____

Play music, then ask each individual in the group to say something about the person next to them. M-31

_____•_•_____

Make choosing a favorite song contingent upon sitting with peers. M-33

Involve the patient in small group discussions, in which all members of the group are encouraged to participate. Suggested topics may focus on the patients themselves, family, work, or future goals. M-31

IS-9 Inappropriate relationships with the opposite sex; inappropriate remarks about sexual topics; asks inappropriate personal questions ($n^3 = 3$; $n^4 = 1$; $n^5 = 4$; 2.26%)

Involve the patient in a coeducational square dance activity with emphasis on appropriate heterosexual interaction (e.g., appropriate touching and verbalization). M-30-40; F-30

Involve the patient in listening-discussion of songs such as "Getting to Know You." Discuss appropriate questions and topics for interactions with females. M-40

IS-10 Self-centeredness; patient has difficulty listening to the problems of others; becomes impatient when sharing attention with other patients ($n^3 = 1$; $n^4 = 2$; $n^5 = 3$; 1.70%)

Have each patient select a song that best describes how they feel. The therapist elicits discussion and feedback from the group members. M-35; F-32

Ask the patient to think of a group member who is interested in people other than him/herself, then select a song which describes the group member. F-30

IS-11 Patient is a loaner who frequently says undesirable things about other patients and staff ($n^3 = 2$; $n^4 = 1$; $n^5 = 3$; 1.70%)

The therapist leads the group in writing lyrics to a familiar song. Each patient must say three nice things about the person on his right. The therapist incorporates the three nice things into the song. M-21; F-21

The therapist reads the lyrics then plays the song, "Just the Way You Are." Follow with a discussion about accepting others in the group. M-35

IS-12 Wears clothing inappropriate for the occasion ($n^3 = 1$; $n^4 = 1$; $n^5 = 2$; 1.13%)

Make attendance at special music programs contingent upon appropriate dress. M-30; F-30

IS-13 Egocentric, childish behavior (e.g., refuses to take turns or to share); does not work well with group ($n^3 = 2$; $n^4 = 0$; $n^5 = 2$; 1.13%)

Present music conditions in which the patient must work and get along with peers. The goal is to foster patient insight into the value of cooperative behavior by having the patient experience the greater benefit of peer acceptance, as opposed to the peer rejection associated with always having one's own way. M-45

The therapist introduces a "mystery song." The patients subsequently play the song in a tone bell ensemble in a cooperative effort to identify the song. M-25

IS-14 Excessive and inappropriate verbalization (e.g., individual is loud and continually talks during the session) ($n^3 = 1$; $n^4 = 1$; $n^5 = 2$; 1.13%)

Arrange conditions to give the patient experience at taking turns talking. For example, let each patient in the group take turns picking out the recording of a song, playing their song for the group, then explaining to the group why they like the song. M-31; F-25

IS-15 Attention seeking ($n^3 = 1$; $n^4 = 1$; $n^5 = 2$; 1.13%)

Involve the patient in a rhythm activity which emphasizes group cooperation rather than individual attention. M-30; F-30

IS-16 Patient exhibits poor group leadership and organizational skills ($n^3 = 1$; $n^4 = 1$; $n^5 = 2$; 1.13%)

Have the patient score a "sound symphony" (percussion instruments) titled "Who Am I?" The patient, using the other group members as performers, will then conduct the symphony. M-35

During group music therapy, provide each group member with the opportunity to lead the group in creative movement to music. F-32

IS-17 Patient frequents barrooms during leisure time; lacks healthy leisure time activities ($n^3 = 1$; $n^4 = 1$; $n^5 = 2$; 1.13%)

Involve the patient in guitar lessons and encourage him to practice during free time. M-33

Give patients an orientation to community activities through field trips to community events such as concerts, plays, and museums. F-30

IS-18 Demonstrates a lack of awareness of others ($n^3 = 1$; $n^4 = 0$; $n^5 = 1$; 00.57%)

Utilize a hand bell performance group (one note per patient) to emphasize working with peers. M-30

IS-19 Difficulty learning names; does not bother to learn the names of persons who bear a close, long term relationship with the patient. ($n^3 = 0$; $n^4 = 1$; $n^5 = 1$; 00.57%)

During music composition, write songs which include the names of the group members and their characteristics. F-28

IS-20 Has difficulty tolerating small groups ($n^3 = 1$; $n^4 = 0$; $n^5 = 1$; 00.57%)

Invite the patient to join the group. Once in the group, give the patient more freedom of choice (e.g., where he sits or which song to sing). M-26

IS-21 Inappropriate relationships with the opposite sex; excessively flirtatious towards male peers ($n^3 = 0$; $n^4 = 1$; $n^5 = 1$; 00.57%)

Involve the patient in structured music therapy sessions (e.g., dance) that teach the patient how to talk with peers without flirting. F-20

IS-22 Aggressive and manipulative ($n^3 = 1$; $n^4 = 0$; $n^5 = 1$; 00.57%)

Present patient-preferred music activities in which mutual consideration and cooperation is required for the success of the activity. M-45

IS-23 Lacks knowledge of how to have fun in a nondestructive manner ($n^3 = 1$; $n^4 = 0$; $n^5 = 1$; 00.57%)

Utilize music (e.g., Music Trivia) and nonmusic games to develop on task socialization, frustration tolerance, and positive leisure activities. M-25

IS-24 Exhibits appropriate behavior at community events ($n^3 = 1$; $n^4 = 0$; $n^5 = 1$; 00.57%)

Take the patients on an outing to a concert in the community. M-85

IS-25 Argues frequently with authority figures ($n^3 = 1$; $n^4 = 0$; $n^5 = 1$; 00.57%)

Involve the patient in drum lessons to sublimate aggression. Also, give the patient experience at relating to leaders in nonthreatening music activities such as chorus and group singing. M-30

IS-26 Interacts with staff but not with peers ($n^3 = 0$; $n^4 = 1$; $n^5 = 1$; 00.57%)

Announce that each patient is going to have to tell something to the group about their neighbor. In the presence of background music, allow each patient to interact with their neighbor about what is to be told. When the music stops, each patient then tells something about their neighbor. F-20

IS-27 Patient becomes impatient and intolerant when another patient chooses a song he doesn't like ($n^3 = 1$; $n^4 = 0$; $n^5 = 1$; 00.57%)

Have each patient choose a song they would like someone else in the group to hear. Discuss the musical characteristics of the song (e.g., dynamics) and the message of the song. M-33

IS-28 Does not participate in leisure activities because of excessive working (e.g., "workaholic") ($n^3 = 1$; $n^4 = 0$; $n^5 = 1$; 00.57%)

Involve the patient in a music exercise group to help develop relaxation techniques. Inform the patient of places that have exercise programs to use after the patient leaves the hospital. M-31

IS-29 Does not participate in leisure activities because they increase stress ($n^3 = 1$; $n^4 = 0$; $n^5 = 1$; 00.57%)

Use a sing-along with songs that identify feelings or leisure activities which reduce stress (e.g., "Bicycle Built for Two"). M-30

IS-30 Patient is withdrawn and passive during one-to-one session with therapist ($n^3 = 1$; $n^4 = 0$; $n^5 = 1$; 00.57%)

Utilize improvisation as a means for individual expression and in nonverbal dialogue with the therapist to increase the patient's awareness of self in relation to others. M-41; F-41

IS-31 Patient stays in bed all day ($n^3 = 1$; $n^4 = 0$; $n^5 = 1$; 00.57%)

Conduct activities on the patient's ward that he may be attracted to, or that might lure him out of bed. Utilize the patient's favorite music in such activities. M-25

IS-32 Patient will not attend group ($n^3 = 1$; $n^4 = 0$; $n^5 = 1$; 00.57%)

Find any special interest in music; agree to play the patient's favorite song. M-25

DRUGS

(Combined, n = 54; 9.98%; Male, n^1 = 23; 42.59%; Female, n^2 = 31; 57.41%

Includes:

D-1.0 SUBSTANCE USE OR ABUSE and MEDICATIONS (Combined, n = 18; 3.33%; Male, n^1 = 8; 44.44%; Female, n^2 = 10; 55.56%)

D-2.0 PHYSICAL WELL BEING (Combined, n = 15; 2.77%; Male, n1 = 5; 33.33%; Female, n^2 = 10; 66.67%)

D-3.0 PHYSICAL COMMUNICATION PROBLEMS (Combined, n = 21; 3.88%; Male, n^1 = 10; 47.62%; Female, n^2 = 11; 52.38%)

PROBLEM

D-1.1 Engages in substance abuse during leisure time; may drink excessively and frequently at local barroom or at home (n^3 = 2; n^4 = 3; n^5 = 5; 27.78%)

MUSIC THERAPY INTERVENTION

Play barroom music (if patient preferred), then have patients discuss the music. The discussion may focus on a lyric/music analysis including whether the lyrics were valid/the meaning or message of the song. M-31

Use lyrics of songs that reflect upon the patient's use of alcohol. Have the patient to verbalize what their life was like before the alcohol abuse and what it is like now. Give the patient a lyric sheet and ask her to listen to the song. F-20

Choose songs for lyric analysis that focus on alcoholism and other addictive problems. F-35

Provide instrumental instruction to develop appropriate leisure interests and as an alternative to substance abuse. M-51; F-51

D-1.2 Patient denies having a substance abuse problem (n^3 = 2; n^4 = 2; n^5 = 4; 16.67%)

From a list of 150 song titles, have the patient select five which relate to themselves. Follow with a listening-discussion session. F-56

During music discussion group, use music with lyrics portraying substance problems (e.g., "Alcohol," the Kinks; "Life in the Fast Lane," the Eagles; "The Pusher Man," Steppen Wolf). This activity may provide a nonthreatening condition for assisting the patient in stating how their problems relate to those in the music. M-31

The patient is given a list of 50 song titles and asked to make two lists of 10 titles each. One list of songs should describe their addiction, and the other list should describe their recovery up to the present. Both lists should show the progression of the addiction and recovery. F-60

Play an appropriate song such as Amy Grant's, "Don't Run Away." Follow with a discussion of life problems the patient may be "running from." M-31

D-1.3 Patient attributes substance abuse to life stress; uses substances for relaxation ($n^3 = 2$; $n^4 = 1$; $n^5 = 3$; 16.67%)

Develop a strategy for reducing stress. Use music relaxation as an alternative to managing stress. Conduct music listening sessions which focus on relaxation with light imagery. Have the patient listen to the music (tapes), imagine a pleasant place, then focus on how he feels afterwards. M-25-30; F-65

D-1.4 Patient lacks awareness of how the pattern of substance abuse has progressed; may be unaware of lost leisure or vocational skills, or lost values. ($n^3 = 1$; $n^4 = 2$; $n^5 = 3$; 16.67%)

Through drawing a record album cover and writing original titles, the patient will describe how life was before treatment, during treatment, and goals for the future. M-85

Teach the patient leisure activities which can be done without the use of drugs. For example, involve the patient in a music exercise class. Focus on increasing self-esteem, self-worth and self-image. F-20

The patient is given a list of ten song titles which can be thought of in terms of values (e.g., values regarding cocaine, friends, faith, etc.). The patient then classifies the values under either "addiction" or "recovery." Follow with a discussion of healthy values. F-60

D-1.5 Patient is reluctant to discuss substance abuse and treatment issues ($n^3 = 1$; $n^4 = 0$; $n^5 = 1$; 5.56%)

Ask the patient to bring a song which describes his addiction. M-85

D-1.6 Manipulates the environment to get their own way, sometimes by being dishonest; may experience guilt. ($n^3 = 1$; $n^4 = 0$; $n^5 = 1$; 5.56%)

Choose songs for lyric analysis that focus on alcoholism and other addictive problems. F-35

D-1.7 Inability to identify coping mechanisms, rehabilitation goals, or to solve problems associated with self-defeating addictive behavior ($n^3 = 0$; $n^4 = 1$; $n^5 = 1$; 5.56%)

Utilizing two lists, each containing 20 song titles, ask the patient to write two short stories. One story, written from the first list, is to describe the patient's own addiction, and the other story, written from the second list, is to describe the patient's recovery. The patient is to incorporate actual song titles into the context of the sentences. F-60

D-1.8 Mourns loss of drug habit ($n^3 = 0$; $n^4 = 1$; $n^5 = 1$; 5.56%)

Use song writing and discussion to help the patient through the mourning. F-31

D-2.1 Absence of daily exercise routine; poor muscle tone ($n^3 = 1$; $n^4 = 1$; $n^5 = 2$; 13.33%)

Involve patient in 20-minute rhythmic exercise routine with prompts, five days per week, or as prescribed. M-30; F-25

D-2.2 Poor personal hygiene ($n^3 = 1$; $n^4 = 1$; $n^5 = 2$; 13.33%)

Make patient's favorite music activity (such as access to the piano or stereo) contingent upon daily bathing. M-30; F-30

D-2.3 Insomnia ($n^3 = 1$; $n^4 = 1$; $n^5 = 2$; 13.33%)

Formulate and record a music/relaxation program for the patient to use PRN (as needed) to decrease insomnia. M-51; F-51

D-2.4 Lack of neuromuscular endurance in upper extremities ($n^3 = 0$; $n^4 = 1$; $n^5 = 1$; 6.67%)

During group improvisation, have the patient improvise five to ten minutes on a variety of percussion instruments. F-25

D-2.5 Poor gross and fine motor coordination ($n^3 = 0$; $n^4 = 1$; $n^5 = 1$; 6.67%)

Assess and treat through various types of music activities (e.g., instrumental lessons, movement to music) F-15

D-2.6 Poor eye-hand coordination (sensory integrative functioning) ($n3 = 1$; $n^4 = 1$; $n^5 = 2$; 13.33%)

During instrumental music improvisation, require the patient to strike the mallet in the center of the xylophone bars. M-30

Play the game, Balloon Toss to Music. Seat the patients in a circle, play some "fun" background music, then ask the patients to take turns "hitting the balloon" to another patient. Because balloons move slowly, this activity allows for delayed reactions characteristic of some patients (e.g., geriatrics). F-30

D-2.6 Vestibular problems (sensory integrative functioning) ($n^3 = 1$; $n^4 = 1$; $n^5 = 2$; 13.33%)

Involve the patient in folk dances which require bending, twisting, and changing directions. See: Schroeder, Block, and Campbell. *Adult Psychiatric Sensory Integration Standardized Assessment* (an occupational therapy assessment). M-26

For problems with vestibular input, use popular dances to give the patient practice at going under the arm of their partner (e.g., two-step Country and Western, part of the Jitterbug). F-31

D-2.6 Lack of proprioceptive feedback (sensory integrative functioning) ($n^3 = 1$; $n^4 = 0$; $n^5 = 1$; 6.67%)

Assess the patient's ability to perceive the beat of the music (See Weikart, *Teaching Folk Dance: Successful Steps*, High/Scope Press, Ypsilanti, MI). Patient performs rhythmic patting to the music first with the hands, then the feet, then by walking to the beat. M-26

D-2.7 Lacks spatial awareness; unaware of position of body in space (sensorimotor) ($n^3 = 0$; $n^4 = 1$; $n^5 = 1$; 6.67%)

Involve the patient in structured dance (e.g., Have a circle dance in which the patients line up holding hands, go backwards 8 to 16 counts, then forward to the starting position). F-31

D-2.8 Lack of diaphragmatic control (from excessive purging associated with eating disorder) ($n^3 = 0$; $n^4 = 1$; $n^5 = 1$; 6.67%)

During choir or individual voice lessons, use vocal exercises that focus on appropriate use of the diaphragm. F-31

D-3.1 Difficulty or inability to verbally communicate with others; unable to maintain conversation; poor communication skills; poor quality of communication during interactions; doesn't communicate coherently; slurs speech; experiences difficulty being understood ($n^3 = 5$; $n^4 = 6$; $n^5 = 11$; 52.38%)

Conduct nonverbal musical call and response activities with the patient (e.g., Therapist plays a musical antecedent at the piano and the patient responds with a musical consequent). M-30

Encourage the patient to sing song lyrics coherently, with good diction. F-25

In a one-to-one session, have the patient sing his thoughts. Gradually expand the song content to permit the patient to tell a complete story. F-20

Have the patients sing and chant familiar song lyrics. F-32

Given Orff instruments, have two patients use the instruments to carry on a conversation with each other. M-30; F-30

Ask the patient to respond musically (nonverbally) on an instrument with the therapist (e.g., during improvisation, the patient solos while the therapist accompanies, or vice versa). F-25

Have patients pass a ball while listening to music. When the music pauses, the patient with the ball verbally responds to a question. M-30

---·•·---

Use musical games that focus on basic communication skills. M-15; F-15

---·•·---

Conduct a "fill in the blank" song writing activity. M-50

---·•·---

Utilize the tape recorder as an assessment and treatment tool. Tape record the patients speech, let the patient listen to the tape recording, formulate and implement speech goals, then evaluate by recording the patient's speech a second time. F-28

D-3.2 Poor nonverbal communication (inappropriate eye contact, affect, and gestures) ($n^3 = 2$; $n^4 = 1$; $n^5 = 3$; 14.29%)

Have the patient use nonverbal communication techniques to direct group Orff improvisation activities. M-30; F-30

Involve the patient in nonverbal conversation by playing music instruments. The music instruments are utilized as the nonverbal communication tool and are played in a "call and response" format. Follow activity with a discussion of appropriate nonverbal cues and communications. M-25

D-3.3 Responds to questions with one word sentences ($n^3 = 1$; $n^4 = 1$; $n^5 = 2$; 9.52%)

During lyric analysis and discussion, have the patient describe what the lyrics mean. M-35; F-32

D-3.4 Exhibits pressured speech ($n^3 = 1$; $n^4 = 1$; $n^5 = 2$; 9.52%)

Use vocal techniques and slow tempi to elicit a slower rate of speaking and more distinct enunciation. M-45; F-37

D-3.5 Patient attempts to communicate but makes irrelevant comments about the topic being discussed. ($n^3 = 1$; $n^4 = 0$; $n^5 = 1$; 4.76%)

During music discussion, redirect patient statements by asking questions related to the topic of the particular lyric analysis. M-31

D-3.6 Poor breath support/control ($n^3 = 1$; $n^4 = 0$; $n^5 = 1$; 4.76%)

Involve the patient in appropriate music therapy activities such as voice or piano lessons. M-15

D-3.7 Patient speaks too softly to be heard ($n^3 = 0$; $n^4 = 1$; $n^5 = 1$; 4.76%)

Have the patient select a song for the group to sing, then loud enough for the group to hear, tell the group the name of the selected song. M-33; F-30

CHAPTER 4

ADOLESCENTS

(N = 156)

CODES

N = Number of music therapy interventions submitted for Adolescents.

n = Number of music therapy interventions submitted for the specific area of assessment. % = Percentage of N.

n^1 = Number of music therapy interventions submitted for each component problem. % = Percentage of n^1.

_____•____ = Separates different types of music therapy interventions (e.g., playing instruments, singing, composing, moving to music, specified behavior modification techniques, other).

   The number(s) after each intervention (e.g., 36) refers to the mean GAF score of the patients for whom the intervention was designed. One score was given by each music therapist specifying the intervention (e.g., "25-30-36" indicates the specific intervention was submitted by three music therapists, and that the intervention is used with patients having the above mean GAF scores).

ASSESSMENT AREA – BEHAVIOR
(n = 11; 7.05%)

PROBLEM

B-1 Lack of assertiveness; unaware of nonverbal, nonassertive body language projected; does not exercise basic classroom rights, obligations, or responsibilities (e.g., the right to think for ones self, the freedom to make mistakes while learning, risking one's opinion); does not state own needs or desires (n^1 = 5; 45.45%)

MUSIC THERAPY INTERVENTION

Give each patient a choice of songs to sing or instrument to play. Each patient must make a selection/decision. 50

Involve the patient in group/individual improvisation on a preferred instrument. 40

_____•_____

Involve the patient in solving cooperation puzzles by using nonverbal communication. 46

_____•_____

Have the patient choose three song titles to be used in confronting oneself, and in confronting a peer on either side of oneself. 50

_____•_____

Role play and compare assertive, aggressive, and passive behavior during group music activities (activities such as creating music, playing instruments, moving to music, and listening to music). 40

B-2 Attention deficit disorder; lack of attention span; attends to tasks only for short durations; lack of concentration (n^1 = 3; 27.27%)

Engage patient for longer periods of time during music activity (e.g., Plays musical composition for longer periods of time without stopping). 50

Give individual music lessons. Structure five minute breaks during the practice time. 31

─────

Have the patient participate in an art project while listening to a favorite song (e.g., Cover a long conference table with a sheet of paper and have the group participate in the drawing of a mural). 36

B-3 Withdraws from social situations (n^1 = 1; 9.09%)

Involve the patient in musical drama. Assign the patient a role which is comfortable and which the patient can tolerate. 36

B-4 Hyperactive; unable to focus (n^1 = 1; 9.09%)

Encourage the patient to focus on one task (e.g., During music lessons, have the patient to focus on one song and one instrument. During choir have the patient focus on one song). 31

B-5 Inability or unwillingness to follow staff directions (n^1 = 1; 9.09%)

Make participation in a socially valued music group contingent upon cooperation with the unit medical teams. 45

AFFECT
(n = 51; 32.69%)

PROBLEM

A-1 Inability to identify/express feelings; states "I don't know" when asked how she or others feel; flat or inappropriate affect; lack of congruity between affect and verbalization (e.g., facial expression, body posture/language, vocal tone and volume doesn't match speech content) (n^1 = 17; 33.33%)

MUSIC THERAPY INTERVENTION

Have the patient identify feelings expressed by the singer/song writer in popular song lyrics. 46-50-50

Conduct a "feeling card" activity in which the patient, given a number of cards, selects the card with the word that matches the feeling projected in the music (e.g., frustration). 46-46

Have the patient bring to the "Music Issues Group," a musical recording which relates to feelings or thoughts about issues chosen by the group for discussion. Encourage the patient to appropriately participate in the discussion. 31

During group discussion, have the patient identify specific feelings or emotions expressed in popular song lyrics. 31

Ask the patient to bring a favorite song to the session, play it for the group, discuss the meaning of the lyrics, and explain why the lyrics are meaningful to the patient. 36

Have the patient listen to instrumental music and identify her own feeling state. 40

Give the patient a list of feelings and ask the patient to choose a song which parallels a feeling from the list. 50

Lay out pictures of faces which project different emotions. Play music which generates strong emotion. Have the patient choose the picture which best represents the emotional quality of the music. Follow with a discussion of the picture, the music, and the emotion. 43

———

Have the patient communicate their present feeling by improvising on an instrument. The patient also may use body language which appropriately expresses their feeling as they improvise (including role playing with instruments). 25-46

Have the patient express any feeling word nonverbally by improvising on rhythm instruments while using body posture representative of the feeling. In the following discussion ask the patient to relate a time when she felt that way. 40-50

———

During a song writing activity, have everyone focus on the theme, "Expressing Myself." 40

Use music composition based on the 12-bar blues pattern. Encourage patients to use lyrics which describe their feelings. 46

A-2 Exhibits anger or rage towards others; overly aggressive; may be destructive to self, others (yelling, fighting), or property (e.g., hitting walls, throwing chairs) ($n^1 = 13$; 25.49%)

Ask the patient to play the drums while maintaining the level of control necessary for maintaining the required tempo, dynamics and other musical characteristics. The goal is to practice maintaining control during periods of frustration, and to provide a constructive outlet for frustration, anger, and other intense emotions. 35-45

During group improvisation on rhythm instruments, ask the group to improvise the meaning of two opposite words (e.g., Improvise "peace," then improvise "chaos"). During group processing, ask the patients to focus on relating to one of the words. 50

Have the patients participate in nonverbal "conversations" with one another by improvising on xylophones or other rhythm instruments. 50

Redirect the patient's behavior toward an awareness of appropriate modes of expression. Begin by expanding the patient's repertoire of emotional responses. For example, during a drum activity, ask the patient to create different rhythms to signify different degrees of feeling/emotion. 35

Give the patient experience at cooperating with other group members in the creation of a desirable musical performance (e.g., Using resonator bells, have the patients improvise on the pentatonic scale). 35

List anger-eliciting situations on a chalkboard (e.g., Your sister just broke your brand new compact disc player). Ask the patient to express on a rhythm instrument how he/she would feel in the situation. Discuss appropriate solutions and the consequences of inappropriate solutions. 43

———————

Have the patient select a song from an album to express the anger being felt. Follow by having the patient identify personal, appropriate alternatives for ventilating the anger. 50

Play two or three popular songs which relate to retaining anger, "blowing up," and appropriately asserting or expressing anger. Follow with a discussion of which technique of expression is most typical of the patient. 50

Ask the patients to bring and share with the group their own "angry" music/songs. Have the patients rank their songs on a continuum of most to least angry. Also, have the patients classify their music/songs as "contributors to" or "relievers from" anger. 50

———————

Make participation in a socially valued music group contingent upon appropriate behavior (i.e., If inappropriate behavior occurs, revoke the patient's group membership for one or two weeks). 45

———————

Using drama and music, have the student act out a stressor (precipitator), followed by positive (adaptive) physical, cognitive, and emotional reactions. Discuss with the student how these reactions felt. 40

———————

Have the patient verbalize impulses related to own feelings, then explore alternative responses (e.g., Have the patient to insert lyrics to a structured song which presents an alternative to the patient's responses). 31

A-3 Experiences stress reactions; may result in difficulties such as sleep disturbance, digestive disorders, anxiety, poor judgment, impulsive behavior, and faulty decision making; poor stress management skills; may interfere with the discussion of painful issues (n^1 = 7; 13.73%)

Employ relaxation, or progressive muscle relaxation training utilizing media and techniques such as music, biofeedback, and video taping. Also use a stress level scale ranging from 1 to 10, and music relaxation with guided imagery. 31-46-43-50

Utilize guided imagery and music (GIM) activities to visualize successful involvement in stressful situations. Promote self-awareness and insight. 50-46

During discussion, assist the patient in discovering acceptable and workable ways, which fit the patient's life style, to cope with stress (e.g., aerobics or other exercise to music; performing music). 31

A-4 Experiences anxiety; may be over ongoing problems, unresolved issues or feelings, internal conflicts, or upcoming event; the anxiety may be reality-based about events such as future placement or discipline; may result in sleep disturbance such as nightmares (n^1 = 4; 7.84%)

Lead the patient in progressive muscle relaxation, and then in guided imagery. Have the patient imagine being in the anxiety-provoking situation, then imagine a positive outcome. Follow with a discussion of how the positive outcome can be a possibility. Encourage the patient to practice the imagery, and assist the patient in choosing background music. 40-50

Develop the patient's musical interests to, at least temporarily, replace the patient's fears. The goal is to use music therapy as a distracter, thereby creating a palliative effect. 36

Teach the patient to use the guitar to accompany breathing exercises (i.e., playing simple relaxing chord progressions, such as F Major ^{7} to C Major ^{7}, to accompany slow, deep breathing). 46

A-5 Lacks self-control; poor impulse control (n^1 = 3; 5.88%)

Employ relaxation training with biofeedback, music response, and key word response. 31

Give piano instruction. The goal is for the patient to begin to experience the self-satisfaction and rewards of self-control by learning to play the piano. 36

Reduce negative comments and sanctions from peers (which may trigger poor impulse control) by improving peer relationships. Involve the patient in a music performance group in which all must work collectively to portray a specific message through the performance (e.g., musical selections/improvisations representing trust and friendship). 36

A-6 Patient has difficulty identifying and verbally sharing feelings related to significant life experiences (e.g., trauma/fears) (n^1 = 2; 3.92%)

Play a song having lyrics related to the patient's trauma/fears. After listening to the song, encourage the patient to share, during group discussion, thoughts, feelings, and symbols that were elicited by the song. 25

Establish patient trust in the music therapist; use songwriting and improvisation activities. 45

A-7 Depressed (n^1 = 2; 3.92%)

During lyric analysis, assist patients in relating the lyrics to their personal lives. Ask the patients to identify similar problems in their lives, then discuss appropriate solutions. 51

Give one-to-one musical instruction. The goal is to increase enthusiasm for life experiences, self-confidence, and peer acceptance through the learning of a socially valued skill. 45

A-8 Suicidal (n^1 = 1; 1.96%)

Ask the patients to bring and share with the group their own "angry" or "depressing" music/songs. Have the patients rank their songs on a continuum of most to least depressing or angry. Also, have the patients classify their music/songs as "contributors to," or "relievers from" depression or anger. 50

A-9 Patient has difficulty expressing positive feelings towards peers (n^1 = 1; 1.96%)

Ask the patient to bring a recording that describes a positive relationship she has with a peer. 20

A-10 Expresses emotions in a variety of socially unacceptable ways (n^1 = 1; 1.96%)

Use songs and improvisation to elicit intense emotions, such as anger and fear. 40

SENSORY
(n = 0; 00.00%)

IMAGERY
(n = 1; 00.64%)

PROBLEM

IM-1 Distorted body image (associated with eating disorder) (n^1 = 1)

MUSIC THERAPY INTERVENTION

Use music with progressive muscle relaxation to help the patient develop body awareness, or a realistic body image. 31

COGNITIVE
(n = 32; 20.51%)

PROBLEM

C-1 Low self-esteem; low sense of values/personal importance causing dysfunctional interpersonal interactions; makes negative self-statements; experiences feelings of worthlessness; lacks self-respect and self-confidence; may exhibit poor eye contact (n^1 = 10; 31.25%)

MUSIC THERAPY INTERVENTION

Reduce negative comments and sanctions from peers (which may produce low self-esteem) by improving peer relationships. Involve the patient in a music performance group in which all must work collectively to portray a specific message through the performance (e.g., musical improvisations/songs representing trust and friendship). 36

Involve the patient in a performance group. Prepare a music performance to be given to peers, therapists, teachers, family, or other significant persons. 50

Give instrumental music instruction. Reinforce realistic musical goals while assisting the patient in identifying unrealistic goals. 46

Provide individualized music therapy sessions focused on learning to play an instrument or song writing. 40

Family involvement is crucial at the high school level. Invite families to musical performances to build self-esteem and to open doors to constructive communication. (Respondent Note: The family has the greatest impact on students. Compared to the family, school and therapy are of secondary importance. The musical performance can be used as a nonthreatening way to involve families.) 50

Emphasize belief in oneself. Give credit to those who try. Help the student to understand there is some success in trying, no matter what the result. Give the students many opportunities to perform. Spare no effort to assure that those who perform are well received. 50

Perform one of the patient's favorite songs on guitar or piano. Ask the patient to listen to the song, then write a parody (new lyrics) of the song. 36

Assist each student in writing their own song. Arrange for each student to receive praise and recognition by playing each student's song at a public performance. 40

Focus on positive rather than negative aspects of behavior. Use individualized music activities which bring out a student's musical strengths. As musical strengths are developed, showcase them! 50

During music therapy, emphasize constructive measures (i.e., correct the behavior, not the child) (Heim Ginott philosophy). The musical/social behavior may need improvement, but the child is accepted unconditionally. 50

C-2   Lacks problem-solving skills; inability to identify a step-by-step procedure for resolving problems; fails to respond to problem-solving cues; fails to recognize apparent solutions to problems; may feel overwhelmed and out of control of self or future ($n^1 = 4$; 12.50%)

Use guided imagery and music relaxation. During guided imagery ask the patient to imagine problem situations and to mentally rehearse being in control. 43-46

Involve the patient in a tone bell ensemble. Provide the patient with tone bell music (therapist constructed music indicating notes to be played and their location on the staff) and direct the group to perform the music. Provide positive reinforcement for correct performances (i.e., correct notes played). Follow with a discussion of processes necessary to the success of the activity. Relate to other life situations. 40

Cut each staff line from a piece of sheet music (complete song), then place the resulting pieces of paper in an envelope. Give the envelope to the patient, asking her to reassemble or reconstruct the music so the therapist can use the music to sing the song. Assist the patient with musical notation and symbols, but encourage the patient to use problem-solving cues inherent in the lyrics (e.g., Do the lyrics rhyme? Are the lyrics logical? Do the lyrics make sense?). 40

C-3 Gives up easily when solving problems; low frustration tolerance; resulting disappointments may lead to inappropriate behavior such as disruptive behavior ($n^1 = 3$; 9.37%)

Involve the patient in the group task of composing or creating a dance to a selected song. Encourage the group members to help one another learn the dance steps. All group members should be involved in the performance of the dance. 40

Involve the patient in activities such as song writing and music improvisation to reduce frustration and inappropriate behavior. 36

———

Present a music activity that requires learning a new skill (e.g., learning new rhythms on percussion instruments). Increase frustration tolerance. 50

C-4 Exhibits paranoid behavior; makes "mountains out of mole hills"; minor incidents considered a threat; does not trust others ($n^1 = 2$; 6.25%)

Concentrate and redirect the patient's attention toward the musical task or activity. The goal is to channel the patient's energy into constructive outlets. 45

———

Have the student participate in a guided imagery experience focused on the issue of trust. 40

C-5 Exhibits "narrow mindedness" causing misunderstandings; does not respond well to suggestions from others, or to constructive criticism ($n^1 = 2$; 6.25%)

Conduct a story-telling activity in which each group member tells a story after/ while listening to nonverbal music. Follow with a discussion of the story content. 36

———

Create compositions (e.g., music, poetry) based on story content derived from guided imagery and music activities. Have students critique the compositions of others; encourage students to accept constructive criticism. 40

C-6 Lacks awareness of, or insight into own personal problems ($n^1 = 2$; 6.25%)

During song writing, write a parody (lyric substitution) about changes that the patient has made and needs to make. Follow with related discussion. 50

———

Using songs reflective of the patient's problems, prompt the patient to relate own behavior, opinions, or problems to those presented in the song. 40

C-7 Poor organizational skills; impaired ability to organize, alphabetize, categorize, or file information or materials related to academic subjects, or school activities in general; inability to prioritize or set goals (n^1 = 2; 6.25%)

Have the students construct a music notebook in which they organize all the music information obtained during music therapy class time. 40

Assist students in establishing and prioritizing individual therapeutic goals which motivate and challenge them. It is very important that students be expected to follow through with (i.e., achieve, or make progress toward) their goals. During music therapy, place a major emphasis on the successful follow-through of music goals to promote positive generalization to other behavior. 50

C-8 Poor conflict identification and resolution skills; experiences ongoing conflict with parents (n^1 = 2; 6.25%)

Discuss music lyrics/ television sitcom situations. Stop the video taped sitcom at predetermined places for a discussion of alternative solutions to problem situations presented in the sitcom. Also discuss the reality of the solutions presented in the song lyrics/sitcom as related to the patient's experiences. 31

Have the patient listen to and discuss the songs, "Father and Son," or "Cats Cradle." Ask the patient to write a letter to the parent with whom there is a conflict describing what the problem is and suggesting some alternatives ways to solve the problem. 40

C-9 Inability to cope with family conflicts (n^1 = 1; 3.12%)

Conduct improvisation with instruments, using the instruments to represent family members engaged in conversation, conflict, and other typical interactions. Follow with a discussion of conflict resolution techniques. 50

C-10 Lacks awareness of one's role in a family, or insight into own family interactions (n^1 = 1; 3.12%)

Have the patient improvise on rhythm instruments, with assistance from others, to show how her family interacts (e.g., appoint one performer to be mother, one to be father, until there is a performer for each member of the family. Improvise typical interactions and scenarios). 50

C-11 Lacks awareness of ones own relationship to peer group (n^1 = 1; 3.12%)

Involve the group in the writing of a musical rap about both the common and individual issues of each group member. 36

C-12 Does not trust therapist; will not honestly communicate with therapist (n^1 = 1; 3.12%)

Trust is the key to success with those who are emotionally disturbed. Until honest communication occurs, there is little or no progress. Only when an emotionally disturbed student feels that you are genuinely there to help will trust and honest communication occur. 50

C-13 Inability to make decisions; does not express preferences, needs, likes or dislikes (n^1 = 1; 3.12%)

Involve the patient in a listening or performance activity. Verbally give the patient feedback about behavioral observations, such as, "I saw you smile and pat your foot during this song. It looked as though you liked it." 46

INTERPERSONAL-SOCIALIZATION
(n = 49; 31.41%) (includes LEISURE SKILLS)

PROBLEM

IS-1 Uncooperative behavior; noncompliant with stated rules and limits; does not follow directions (e.g., "Stay in your chair," "Stay on task," "Work quietly," "Be nice to others," "Finish your work on time," "Raise your hand before speaking"); refuses to take turns, share or to compromise; conduct disorder; exhibits inappropriate behavior both on and off hospital/school grounds (n^1 = 13; 26.53%)

MUSIC THERAPY INTERVENTION

Involve the patient in an instrumental performance group. Assign responsibilities (e.g., musical roles) so each patient's cooperation is dependent upon group success. 51

Involve the patient in activities that require the sharing of leadership (e.g., improvisation). 50

Involve the patient in group improvisation activities. 40

During a xylophone improvisational activity give each patient a tone bar. Ask the group to follow (imitate) the musical characteristics of the designated leader's improvisation (e.g., imitate dynamics and tempo). 35

During a drum activity, ask the patients to pass the drum around the group, and for each patient to play a different rhythm. 35

———

Involve the patient in a highly structured group musical game with contingent music listening as the reward for winners (e.g., Use musical games such as Crosswords, lyric puzzles, and Music Trivia which focus on team work and cooperation). 40-50

Make attendance at music sessions (singing, listening to music, moving to music, creating music, playing instruments) contingent upon earning points in the "classroom discipline point system." 40

Give the group a stack of recordings and ask them to choose two selections of music they would like to hear. 20

Make attending a local performance or concert contingent upon appropriate behavior. 20

Have the patients work together on a project such as a musical collage. 20

Involve the patient in dance and rhythmic exercise groups which require listening to, and then following directions. 36

Involve the student in lyric interpretation leading to a discussion of ineffective and effective coping techniques. 40

IS-2 Lacks awareness of self or others; detached; poor peer relationships; does not interact appropriately with peers (e.g., does not give or receive positive comments; excessively negative); lacks respect for others; has difficulty making friends; distances others through sarcasm, anger, and other destructive defenses ($n^1 = 12$; 24.49%)

Involve the patient in group rehearsals and the subsequent performance of a song. 40

During performance group, redirect patient comments such as "I Like the way that sounds" to "[Patient's name] played well." Discuss reactions of peers to positive/negative statements. 46

Provide experience at supporting others by involving the patient in "supported solos" during group improvisation. The patient will demonstrate the ability to both accompany other patients and the ability to take solos while being accompanied. Monitor the patient's ability to take both leader and follower roles. 50

Do the activity, "Song Title Feedback Fan." Each patient takes turns selecting a song title representative of each group member. The song titles are then assembled into the shape of a paper fan, and discussed with each group member. 50

Conduct lyric discussions about songs which identify (1) destructive defenses, and (2) positive self-protection in relationships. 40

Involve the patient in activities which require working with group members toward common goals, or emphasizing or utilizing the strengths of each member (e.g., video projects involving music or drama). 31

Involve the patient in group activities such as making a music video, putting on a radio show (e.g., interviewing), and music composition (song statement). 46

Involve the patient in group activities such as playing instruments, learning popular songs, lyric analysis with discussion, drawing to music, lyric writing, and music appreciation (contrasting popular artists). Emphasize appropriate interaction (e.g., appropriate language, taking turns, complimenting peers, positive self-statements). 51-50

Involve the patient in writing and performing song parodies (rewriting lyrics), and in sharing information about each group member. 40

Involve the patient in activities that provide unique individual attention, such as a talent show. 36

Involve the patient in group music activities requiring interaction through touch, verbalization, and movement. 50

IS-3 Withdrawn; does not share thoughts, feelings, or interests; does not ask or answer questions; does not communicate with others; isolates self ($n^1 = 9$; 18.37%)

During music listening, play music which was popular in past decades. Ask the students to identify the decade in which the music was popular, to identify the instrumentation, and to discuss societal issues which were prevalent when the music was popular (i.e., Discuss issues of the 1950s, '60s, '70s, and '80s after listening to music of the same era). 40

Ask students to contribute to history charts, or a music notebook, showing aspects of life in the 1950s, '60s, '70s, and '80s. Ask them to contribute recorded music, books, videos, and pictures. 40

Ask each group member to bring to the next session a recording of a favorite song, to play it for the group, and to briefly describe the music, the performer, and any other points of interest about the recording. 50

Ask the patient to choose songs to play for the group which communicate messages to the group. After the group listens to the song, follow with a discussion and feedback about what the group heard communicated. 40

During "Music Exploration," ask the patients to bring information on a chosen music topic to the next meeting. At the next meeting, have the patients discuss the information they found on the music topic. Plan a community outing to observe the performance of the music (e.g., An example topic might be "Recorded Music." At the next session have the patients discuss how music is recorded and work on a group song to record. Plan to visit a recording studio and observe the studio musicians). 31

Involve the group in the writing of a canon which uses names of the group members. Encourage the group members to work together so the canon can be performed successfully. 43

Have the patients express their own ideas by filling in the blanks when using a "fill in the blanks" music composition activity (e.g., the patient completes open, or incomplete lyrical statements). 50

Encourage group involvement by utilizing activities such as playing instruments, group singing, and musical games. Assign an individual part in a performance ensemble (per patient ability). Do not try to force conversation. Gradually add more discussion requirements. 31-46

IS-4 | Inappropriately uses leisure time; lacks knowledge of community-based leisure activities available to students; spends leisure time with gangs ($n^1 = 6$; 12.24%)

Give instruction in how to teach one's self to play a music instrument (e.g., guitar, keyboard). Give the necessary materials to the patient and check weekly for progress and questions. Encourage home practice. 31-46-40

Give music lessons; involve the patient in the school band or orchestra, or in other community activities. 46

Expand music preferences to include a variety of styles. Musical preferences can be developed during music listening, music theory, and instrumental and vocal instruction. 46

Expand knowledge of arts activities in the community; discuss arts events listed in the newspaper; take weekly field trips to arts events. 40

Teach musical games, such as Instrument Pictionary, Name That Tune, and Musical Bingo. 43

IS-5 | Does not/lacks motivation to engage in leisure activities ($n^1 = 3$; 6.12%)

Assess leisure activity by having the patients share their leisure experiences. Ask each patient to bring a song to the next group meeting which describes their leisure activity, hobby, or interests. 20

Encourage the patient to volunteer to assist in providing programming and running the hospital radio station. To develop music involvement, ask the patient to volunteer for "available positions in music" which are needed for music programming. 31

Involve the patient in musical games such as Music Concentration. 30

IS-6 Does not/uninterested in listening to the desires and needs of others; interrupts peers when they are speaking or performing; does not respect the opinions of others (n^1 = 2; 4.08%)

During music listening assign each group member a time to play their preferred music for the rest of the group. Make listening to and respecting each group member's right to play their music contingent upon getting a time to play one's own preferred music for the group (i.e., the patient who does not listen or participate appropriately loses his/her turn). 45

Have the students work together to create a music video (including taping and editing) with original script/lyrics and musical accompaniment. 40

IS-7 Excessive fear of rejection; rejects others to avoid being rejected; excessive fear of not being accepted by others (n^1 = 1; 2.04%)

Use round robin story telling. In the presence of background program music, give each patient three minutes to tell a story based on the music. After three minutes, ask a second patient to continue the story where the first patient left off. Each patient's participation is vital to the success of the activity. 43

IS-8 Uses inappropriate behavior as a means to gain attention (n^1 = 1; 2.04%)

Reinforce patients who display appropriate behavior during the music therapy session (e.g., give first choice of instrument). 43

IS-9 Does not share or take turns (n^1 = 1; 2.04%)

Involve the patient in the playing of games in which the winner gets first chance, second chance, or third chance. 45

IS-10 Poor leadership skills; does not take the initiative (n^1 = 1; 2.04%)

During an instrumental or vocal call and response activity give each student a chance to be the leader. 40

DRUGS

(n = 12; 7.69%)

Includes:

D-1.0 SUBSTANCE USE OR ABUSE

D-2.0 MEDICATIONS (no problems submitted)

D-3.0 PHYSICAL WELL BEING (no problems submitted)

PROBLEM

D-1.1 Lacks knowledge of the effects of chemicals upon physical and psychological functioning; unaware of or denies chemical dependency or loss of self-control (n^1 = 4; 33.33%)

MUSIC THERAPY INTERVENTION

Discuss and interpret the lyrics of songs such as "Life In The Fast Lane" and "I'm Your Pusher." Encourage the patients to share their feelings/experiences during the discussion. Role play negative behaviors and consequences to increase self-awareness. 20-46

Have the patients write about their abuse, getting their ideas from a list of song titles selected by the therapist and based upon the music preferences of the patients. 20

Ask the patient to identify physical/psychological cravings present (elicited) when listening to music they formerly associated with the use of chemicals (e.g., "heavy metal" rock music). 50

D-1.2 Uses substances regularly; may be a maladaptive coping mechanism for stress or unpleasant situations; may use drugs for recreation (n^1 = 3; 25.00%)

CTD (Clinical Training Director) note: Adolescents at this facility do not necessarily use the 12-step program. I have found a performance type of group to be more beneficial for our adolescents than a verbal/insight oriented group. 46

Replace recreational substance abuse with individual instrumental lessons. 43

Teach relaxation techniques as a type of chemical-free stress management. 50

D-1.3 Uses substances to "control" behavior and to block feelings (to numb affect) (n^1 = 2; 16.67%)

Use lyric analysis and discussion to assist the patient in identifying and expressing feelings without drug use. 40

Have the patient identify feeling in music using an adjective checklist. 31

D-1.4 Experiences severe depression while mourning the loss of the substance ($n^1 = 1$; 8.33%)

Utilize song writing to assist the patient in getting in touch with rehabilitation goals and in mourning the loss. 31

D-1.5 Patient links own identity to substance abuse (i.e., "being a druggie") ($n^1 = 1$; 8.33%)

Explore personal identity as it relates to music preferences, including the inter-relation of music and substance abuse (i.e., lyrics which discuss drug use). 40

D-1.6 Lack of diaphragmatic control (from excessive purging associated with eating disorder) ($n^1 = 1$; 8.33%)

During choir or individual voice lessons, use vocal exercises that focus on appropriate use of the diaphragm. 31

CHAPTER 5

CHILDREN

(N = 122)

CODES

N = Number of music therapy interventions submitted for Children.

n = Number of music therapy interventions submitted for the specific area of assessment. % = Percentage of N.

n^1 = Number of music therapy interventions submitted for each component problem. % = Percentage of n^1.

———··——— = Separates different types of music therapy interventions (e.g., playing instruments, singing, composing, moving to music, specified behavior modification techniques, other).

The number(s) after each intervention (e.g., 36) refers to the mean GAF score of the patients for whom the intervention was designed. One score was given by each music therapist specifying the intervention (e.g., "25-30-36" indicates the specific intervention was submitted by three music therapists, and that the intervention is used with patients having the above mean GAF scores).

ASSESSMENT AREA – BEHAVIOR
(n = 18; 14.75%)

PROBLEM

B-1 Unassertive; does not express own needs; lacks inquiry skills (observe for anxiety or fears, evasiveness, or preoccupations); unable to express true feelings or opinions independent of peer pressure; feels compelled to agree with "the right" answer, or the answer given by peers (n^1 = 6; 33.33%)

MUSIC THERAPY INTERVENTION

Ask the patient to use pictures or signs to indicate choice of instrument to use during music activity. 20

Ask the patient to conduct the group. Give the patient a conductor's baton, and the group members a variety of instruments. Ask the patient conducting to communicate dynamics, tempo and when the music should start or stop. 36

After playing a song in a small ensemble, ask the patient to talk about what she experienced while playing. 46

———··———

Encourage the patient to actively participate by expressing own spontaneous feelings and opinions when prompted during song discussion. 36

———··———

When discussing problem solving or conflict situations, each patient will take turns stating opinions which agree and differ from those stated by the majority of patients. 36

Play musical games which require the patient to ask questions. 36

B-2 Attention deficit; lack of attention span; distracted by internal/external stimuli; does not maintain interest in task; poor concentration skills (n^1 = 5; 27.78%)

During singing activities, encourage the child to finish singing the song while maintaining a rhythmic beat. 56

Given the lyrics of a song, ask the staff or a patient to read the lyrics. Observe whether each patient remains seated, listens quietly, and talks appropriately (i.e., only when asked). 50

Reinforce in-seat behavior using instrument play activities. 36

Require that the patient complete the assigned task before moving on to another task/comment. 36

Arrange the musical task to provide incentive for focus of attention and completion. 45

B-3 Does not take turns (e.g., impulsively grabs instrument) (n^1 = 3; 16.67%)

Write a list of 11 roles coveted by the children (e.g., leading the group in the playing of instruments). Assign a number (2 through 12) to each role, so that when two die are rolled, the number appearing on the die is also the number of a role. Each child then takes turns rolling the dye and assuming the role. 40

Involve the patient in a rhythm band in which each person changes instruments upon cue. 56

Utilize a song which requires everyone to take turns. Encourage the patient to take turns communicating to the group. 36

B-4 Hits peers (n^1 = 3; 16.67%)

Involve the patient in a puppet show focused on a musical drama about feelings. 56

Encourage appropriate use of rhythm sticks (i.e., doesn't hit peers). 50

Make participation in coveted music therapy activity contingent upon keeping hands, feet, and objects to self. 40

B-5   Exhibits poor eye contact (n^1 = 1; 5.56%)

Sing the child's name in a song. The therapist presents own hands before the child and offers to do a push and pull activity. 45

AFFECT
(n = 10; 8.20%)

PROBLEM

A-1   Impaired ability to Identify/expresses feelings; demonstrates affect inappropriate to mood; facial expression may be flat, blunt, labile, or sad; poor vocabulary of feeling words (n^1 = 10; 100.00%)

MUSIC THERAPY INTERVENTION

Give the patient a set of cards, each card having the drawing of a person's face depicting a specific emotion (e.g., happy, sad, mad). Ask the patient to identify the feeling depicted, and how the feeling is frequently expressed. Have the patient then select an instrument and nonverbally express the same feeling using the instrument, or select a song that correlates with the emotion. (Note: A variation of this activity is to first, have the patients draw facial features that express basic emotions, then follow with the above music activities). 33-40

Give instruments to the group then ask the group to play a specific feeling (e.g., the therapist says "Lets sound sad." The children then play how they think sad should sound.). Follow with a discussion of what makes each child feel sad. 36

Ask the patients to express specific feelings by playing rhythm instruments. Observe for appropriate feeling response. 86

———•+•———

Have the group sing the song, "If You're Happy and You Know It" while moving as if they are happy. Vary the activity to elicit different emotions by changing the lyrics (e.g., "If you're sad and you know it...") and the accompanying movements. 40

Sing the peekaboo song using a soft scarf to hide the therapist's face from the patient. At the end of the song pull the scarf away and say "boo!" Note the quality of the patient's affective response. 45

———•+•———

Have the patients listen to short musical selections, then indicate through facial expressions how they felt while listening. Vary the activity by having patients report verbally how they felt while listening. 50

Have the patient listen to a variety of musical styles. Include music which the patient both prefers and does not prefer. Ask the patient to discuss her preferences. 46

———————

Play the game Music Bingo to nonverbal music. 56

Observe whether the patient shows appropriate affective response (e.g., laughter, humor, smiling, anticipation) during music activities. 20

SENSORY
(n = 6; 4.92%)

PROBLEM

S-1   Lacks auditory sequential memory (listening, auditory perception) (n^1 = 3; 50.00%)

MUSIC THERAPY INTERVENTION

Assess the patient's ability to follow sequential steps given aurally. Given instruction on how to play rhythm instruments, present the patient with various types and numbers of rhythm instruments. Play the instruments in sequential order and ask the patient to repeat the sequence (e.g., First strike the drum, then the cymbal, and then the resonator bell. Ask the patient to imitate). 36

———————

Conduct music activities in which children must listen to, then follow directions. 50

———————

Have the patient listen to age-appropriate music, then tell about the musical characteristics, such as form and instrumentation. 40

S-2   Lacks auditory discrimination skills (listening, auditory perception) (n^1 = 3; 50.00%)

First assess the ability to discriminate gross musical sounds (e.g., discriminates the sound of a drum from a piano). Next assess the ability to make finer auditory discriminations, such as speech sounds (e.g., discriminates male from female voice, discriminates words and syllables) and more subtle music sounds. 36

Have the patient listen to age-appropriate music, then tell about the musical characteristics, such as form and instrumentation. 40

Utilize music listening activities to teach concepts such as start and stop, loud and quiet, and fast and slow. Have patients match the concept with the type of music heard (e.g., Patient says "fast" when fast music is played and "slow" when slow music is played. Also, have patients identify concepts using alternative communication techniques (i.e., signs, picture symbol cards). 20

IMAGERY
(n = 2; 1.64%)

PROBLEM

IM-1 Inability to experience thoughts when attempting to relax (n^1 = 1; 50.00%)

MUSIC THERAPY INTERVENTION

Have the patient listen to quiet, relaxing music without talking, then give verbal feedback about their experience. 50

IM-2 Inability to use imagination to develop stories (n^1 = 1; 50.00%)

Have the patients listen to quiet music as they draw/express themselves on paper. 50

COGNITIVE
(n = 18; 14.75%)

PROBLEM

C-1 Difficulty following directions; consider the difficulty of the instructions, the physical ability to follow directions, retention ability, and the ability to accept or listen to instructions (n^1 = 6; 33.33%)

MUSIC THERAPY INTERVENTION

Involve the patient in instrumental tasks, such as learning a pattern on a xylophone, or a rhythmic pattern on the drum. 46

Have the patients develop a code language, communicated with rhythm instruments. After the code is developed, divide the patients into two groups, then let each group take turns sending messages (directives) to the other group. When a group receives a directive, they must follow the directive by performing the task requested in the directive. 40

During group singing, require the patient to listen for page numbers to be announced, then turn to the correct page. 33

During group singing, ask the patient to find the page number of a song by looking in the table of contents. Also, give commands such as "Look in the back of the book," Look in the front of the book," Look at the top of the page," and "Look at the bottom of the page." 33

Present songs containing one-step, two-step, and multistep directions (e.g., body action songs such as "clap your hands, pat your knees, then stomp your feet" to the tune "If You're Happy and You Know It," movement to music, circle or other simple dances). 45

—————·—·———

Make raising one's hand before speaking contingent upon choice of music instrument or song. 40

C-2 Lacks directionality and spatial concepts (n^1 = 3; 16.67%)

Use music activities designed to teach concepts such as right from left, and up from down [See: W. Janiak (1978). *Songs for Music Therapy*]. 36

Observe spatial awareness in relation to objects in the room by having the patient walk around the outer perimeter of a circle of chairs during a music activity. 20

Observe spatial awareness in relation to other patients by asking the patient to line up next to/behind/in front of another patient for music movement activities. 20

C-3 Low self-esteem; negative self-concept; makes negative self-statements; may refuse to participate in group activities (n^1 = 2; 11.11%)

When assessing the success of music accomplishments, record the number of positive self-statements and positive peer statements which are made independent of prompts. 36

—————·—·———

Play the game, Music Charades in which patients take turns creatively moving to nonverbal music, as the other patients try to guess the feeling being expressed. The goal is increased self-confidence through successful group participation. 56

C-4 Observe method and quality of approach to tasks (e.g., disorganized vs. goal directed; fast without concern for quality vs. slow and deliberate; gives up easily vs. perseverance; inaccurate vs. accurate) (n^1 = 1; 5.56%)

Teach the patient to perform a song on an instrument, such as using the autoharp to provide a chordal accompaniment, or playing an ostinato pattern on the marimba. 46

C-5 Manipulates using intimidation (makes derogatory comments to peers to effect specific behavior) (n^1 = 1; 5.56%)

During song writing, teach the sharing of concepts by singing the children's thoughts, feelings, and ideas about appropriate ways of meeting one's needs. 56

C-6 Lacks temporal or time concepts ($n^1 = 1$; 5.56%)

Use music activities designed to teach time skills [See: Cary L. Reichard & Dennis B. Blackburn (1973). *Music Based Instruction for the Exceptional Child*]. 36

C-7 Lacks money concepts ($n^1 = 1$; 5.56%)

Use music activities designed to teach money concepts [See: Cary L. Reichard & Dennis B. Blackburn (1973). *Music Based Instruction for the Exceptional Child*]. 36

C-8 Cannot recall letters of the alphabet ($n^1 = 1$; 5.56%)

Play games such as Musical Anagrams (Schulberg, 1981). Fill in blanks on the blackboard to spell the name of a favorite singer or instrument. Sing a song about the letters of the alphabet (e.g., "The Alphabet Song"), stopping the song at various points and asking a patient to point to the letter being sung. 33

C-9 Poor counting skills; may not remember correct numerical sequence ($n^1 = 1$; 5.56%)

Ask the patient to find a specific page number in a songbook. 33

C-10 Poor reading and writing skills ($n^1 = 1$; 5.56%)

Assign the patient to use the school library to compile a music notebook about music of other lands. 40

INTERPERSONAL-SOCIALIZATION
($n = 32$; 26.23%)

PROBLEM

IS-1 Exhibits disruptive or socially inappropriate behavior; may exhibit disruptive outbursts to attract attention; breaks rules; may make negative comments to peers resulting in rejection by peers; does not make constructive suggestions ($n^1 = 9$; 28.13%)

MUSIC THERAPY INTERVENTION

Make music therapy activities such as singing, listening, moving, creating music, and playing instruments contingent upon classroom discipline. Utilize a point system (Various methods are used: (1) Write each patient's name on a large poster and tack the poster to the wall. Next to each name place five plastic push pins, each representing a certain number of minutes the patient may spend in a music activity. Pull a pin for each occurrence of inappropriate behavior (response cost). (2) Same as "1" except give pins for appropriate behavior and pull pins for inappropriate behavior. (3) Have the patient carry a chart. The chart must be initialed by all or a predetermined number of the patient's teachers, verifying good classroom behavior, in order to participate in music activities). 40

During general music therapy activities, if a patient fails to demonstrate desired behavior, initiate a step-wise discipline procedure beginning with a "stop and think" verbal reminder, followed by removal from the activity, then from the group if the behavior does not comply. 40

Make each child being the conductor for her favorite song contingent upon appropriate behavior. 56

Make good grades in music contingent upon appropriate participation in music activities. Give check marks for positive behavior. 50

During song lyric discussion involving staff and patients, reinforce constructive criticism, suggestions, and interpretations about the content of the song lyrics. 50

Ask the patients to remain quiet while listening to a selection of music. Observe responses. 86

Involve the patient in as many group music activities as possible, particularly those requiring interpersonal interaction. 36

Ask the patients to assist in putting together a musical collage of a group of musical artists. Observe for disruptive behavior. 86

Involve the patient in creative marching to upbeat nonverbal music. 56

IS-2 Withdrawn; minimal or no verbal interaction; does not participate in group activities; avoids interaction with peers; shy; timid; not interested in peers (n^1 = 8; 25.00%)

Use a music rhythm band to encourage nonverbal interaction. 56

Have the patient repeat a rhythmic pattern on the claves. Increase the difficulty of the rhythm. Switch roles; have the patient initiate the rhythm pattern and the therapist imitate. 46

Have the patient initiate appropriate verbal interaction with another patient during routine interactive music activities (e.g., "Do you want the drum?" "Will you be my partner?" "Hold the autoharp while I strum."). 20

Ask each patient to bring a song that describes their relationship with a peer to the music therapy session. Ask each patient to play the song, then discuss their relationship with the peer. 86

Ask the patient to choose a song that a peer would enjoy. 33

———·•·———

Involve the patient in as many group music activities as possible. 20-36

———·•·———

Encourage the patient to interact positively with peers during a greeting song activity. 36

IS-3   Uncooperative with adults and peers; argues with peers; does not negotiate or compromise (n^1 = 7; 21.88%)

Have the patient repeat a rhythmic pattern on the claves. Increase the difficulty of the rhythm. Switch roles; have the patient initiate the rhythm pattern and the therapist imitate. Note quality of interaction (e.g., fearful, comfortable, domineering, defensive) with adults/authority figures. 46

Involve the patient in ensemble tasks such as Orff instrumental activities. Observe for appropriate peer interactions (e.g., mutuality in interactions, problem solving). 46

Play the Musical Search Game: (1) Let instrumental sounds represent movement cues (e.g., The sound of the tambourine means to walk forward; the sound of the maracas means to turn; a loud drum beat means the searcher is getting closer to the hidden object; a soft drum beat means the searcher is going away from the hidden object; the sound of a high pitched rhythm instrument (triangle, high pitched tone or xylophone bar) means to reach up; the sound of a low pitched rhythm instrument (low pitched tone or xylophone bar or bass drum) means to reach down. (2) Choose a patient to be the searcher, blindfold the searcher, and tell the searcher that her peers will provide "hints" (cues) for finding the hidden object by playing the rhythm instruments. An adult or another peer may act as "Sound Department Director," specifying when each instrument is to be played (NOTE: This role may be eliminated as patients gain experience with the game). 36

Have the patients assist one another with the construction of music instruments. Observe social behavior. 86

———·•·———

Divide the patients into groups of three or four. Give each group a stack of recordings and ask them to select three songs they would like to hear. 86

Have the patient work with a peer in choosing a song that suits both of them. 33

———·•·———

Involve the patient in a music activity which requires cooperation/teamwork with a peer. Observe whether the patient responds appropriately to other patients' nonverbal and verbal socialization efforts. 20

IS-4 Does not share (n^1 = 4; 12.50%)

Ask the patient to equally divide the time that she and her peers get to play an instrument. 50

Give two patients a set of bongos or a large drum and ask them to play the drum together while following the directives of the song (e.g., "Play the drum soft," "Play the drum loud"); have the children share other rhythm instruments. 45-50

Involve the children in the playing of musical games in which they must share or take turns. 50

IS-5 Interrupts the speaker and activity by extraneous talking (n^1 = 1; 3.13%)

Reinforce task behavior through active participation in a pentatonic ensemble. Use eye contact to communicate when each individual is to start and stop playing her instrument. 36

IS-6 Inaudible speaking voice (n^1 = 1; 3.13%)

During group singing, ask the patient to announce, loud enough for the group to hear, a song choice to the group. 33

IS-7 Lacks leadership skills (n^1 = 1; 3.13%)

Give the child experience at assuming and maintaining a leadership role during rhythm instrument activities. Give the child "stop" and "go" signs, asking her to signal the group when to start playing and when to stop playing their instruments. 45

IS-8 Does not express or respond to greetings or closings (i.e., good-byes) (n^1 = 1; 3.13%)

Use a greeting song (e.g., "Hello Song") at the beginning of the session and a good-bye song (e.g., Good-bye patient's name to the tune of "Good Night Ladies") at the end of the session. Prompt verbal hellos and good-byes using appropriate gestures (e.g., hand shaking) (See: Konnie K. Saliba, *Good Morning Songs & Wake-Up Games*). 45

DRUGS
(n = 18; 14.75%)

Includes:

D-1.0 PHYSICAL WELL BEING

D-2.0 PHYSICAL COMMUNICATION PROBLEMS

D-3.0 SUBSTANCE ABUSE and MEDICATIONS (No problems submitted)

PROBLEM

D-1.1 Impaired gross motor coordination; difficulty performing basic movement tasks; awkward when attempting common movements such as walking; runs into people when in a group (n^1 = 5; 28.78%)

MUSIC THERAPY INTERVENTION

Involve the patient in music movement activities which incorporate skills such as walking, skipping, hopping, and marching. Model the movements using songs which specify the type of movement in the lyrics (e.g., W. Janiak, *Songs for Music Therapy*, "Hop Like a Bunny"). 46

During creative movement to music, have the patient mirror movements and lead movements for peers. 36

Involve the patient in music activities such as mirroring movements, imitating object/animal movement (e.g., The patients walk like a turkey after doing the Thanksgiving turkey chant [C. Bitcon, *Alike and Different*]), moving to various tempi, and working with a partner or the group in movement tasks. 40

Involve the children in musical games involving gross motor movements. 50

Beat a mano drum while the patients walk to the beat. Ask the patients to adjust their walking pace when the beat is varied. Play the drum in different positions (i.e., right-side-up, up-side-down, sideways), letting each position represent a different way to walk (i.e., forward, backward, sideways). 36

D-1.2 Lacks finger dexterity (fine motor) (n^1 = 2; 11.11%)

Give individual keyboard instruction emphasizing melodies and finger exercises utilizing all five fingers. Encourage independent finger movement. 36-51

D-1.3 Has difficulty grasping or manipulating utensils; does not utilize fine motor skills commensurate with age level; impaired grasp function (e.g., palmer, pincer) (n^1 = 2; 11.11%)

Involve the patient in instrumental music activities (e.g., pushing buttons to play the autoharp, grasping a guitar/autoharp pick, playing the finger cymbals, finger strums on the guitar, using mallets to play tone bars). 45-46

D-1.4 Lacks eye-hand motor coordination ($n^1 = 2$; 11.11%)

Have the patients listen to a recorded performance of "Bell Dance." Replay the recording and ask the patients to play along using resonator bells. 50

Ask the patients to listen to a recording of "To The Music I." Replay the recording and ask the patients to clap when the command to clap is given in the lyrics (claps on cue). Note correct/incorrect clapping. 50

D-1.5 Often drops objects causing disruptions to others and embarrassment to self ($n^1 = 1$; 5.55%)

Involve the patient in instrumental activities. Encourage the patient to hold the instrument. 40

D-2.1 Cannot describe objects, feelings, or situations; lacks descriptive skills; note whether verbal quality is logical, coherent, and concrete vs. abstract, and whether language development is appropriate for age ($n^1 = 2$; 11.11%)

Ask the patient to listen to the "words" of a song and then tell what took place in the song. 46

Tell or give the patient several objects, feelings, or situations and ask the patient to describe them without mentioning the name of the object, feeling, or situation. Encourage the patient's search for descriptive qualities; play "detective" games. 36

D-2.2 Impaired ability to Imitate speech or nonspeech sounds ($n^1 = 1$; 5.55%)

Use songs such as "Old MacDonald" and "The Wheels on the Bus" to elicit the imitation of animal sounds, sounds of environmental objects (i.e., the bus), and speech sounds (song lyrics). 45

D-2.3 Exhibits explosive rather than a comfortable level of speech ($n^1 = 1$; 5.55%)

Engage the patients in group singing, giving each member a solo. 56

D-2.4 Poor speech articulation ($n^1 = 1$; 5.55%)

Engage the patient in the singing of songs; chant the lyrics; emphasize clear pronunciation. 40

D-2.5 Impaired receptive language ability; poor comprehension ($n^1 = 1$; 5.55%)

Discuss the meaning of song lyrics; critique musical performances. 40

CHAPTER **6**

ADULTS – MUSIC BEHAVIOR

(Combined, N = 364; Male, N^1 = 147; 40.39% Female, N^2 = 217; 59.62%)

ASSESSMENT AREA – LISTENING TO MUSIC
(Combined, n = 112; 30.77%; Male, n^1 = 47; 41.96%; Female, n^2 = 65; 58.04%)

BEHAVIOR

L-1 Demonstrates musical preferences (n^3 = 12; n^4 = 24; n^5 = 36; 32.14%)

MUSIC THERAPY INTERVENTION

When asked, the patient will express preference for a favorite music style, performer, or composer. NOTE: The therapist may wish to follow up by playing the preferred song for the patient and inviting the patient to join in the singing of the lyrics. M-25-30-30-32; F-26-30-31-35-36-39-50-65

Given a collection of recordings or albums, the patient will select a song to play for the group (e.g., Given a table with a stack of twenty albums, ask the patient to go to the table and pick an album to play for the group; an alternative is to ask the patient to bring a recording from her personal record collection, or to select a recording from the record library in the music therapy room). Follow with lyric interpretation and discussion. THERAPIST NOTE: If the patient does not respond to this procedure in a group situation, repeat the procedure in an individualized or one-to-one session with the patient. Songs used should have recovery themes. F-25-30-31-39-60

Involve the patient in a discussion of musical preferences. Assign the patient to research the topic of music in the hospital library, then share the resulting information with the group. Assign the patient to listen to the music of a particular composer, to gather historical information about the composer, and then to present to the group an oral report (with recorded musical examples) about the style of the composer. M-35; F-41-37

Ask the patient to identify music-related activities he or she engages in at home (e.g., listening to records, watching musicals on television, listening to music on the radio, visiting music stores, going to concerts and recitals). M-40; F-35

Ask the patient to bring recordings of and information about one of their preferred musical artists to present to the group. M-85; F-31

During music listening, ask the patients to rate their preference for the songs played. Give each patient the opportunity to share their music ratings with others (e.g., Play "Rate a Record" in which various musical selections are played and each patient rates their preference for each selection using a 10-point scale). M-30; F-65

Show the patient the catalogued collection of recordings and ask him to choose a recording of his favorite artist for music listening. Encourage the patient to talk about his favorite recordings or albums. M-40

Make a music preferences tape in which many styles of music are represented. Play the tape and ask the patient to say "yes" or "no" to indicate her preference for each style of music. F-25

Ask the group to rank given musical compositions in the order they are to be played. Encourage group discussion of the aspects of each composition (e.g., positive aspects versus negative aspects). M-35

Administer a questionnaire that requires the patient to identify the type of music she listens to when she is happy, the type she listens to when she is sad, and what she likes best about the music (e.g., may include comments about the lyrics, melody, beat, or tempo). F-56

Given a list of 30 songs, the patient will select one song for the group to sing. M-35

Have each patient select a song to play for the group. After the group has listened attentively to each song, discuss the song. Have the group rank in order the songs from most preferred to least preferred. F-37

Encourage the patient to independently initiate music listening during listening session and/or leisure time. M-30

Include questions on the assessment questionnaire to identify the patient's preferred modality (e.g., art, music, dance, movement, recreation) for addressing treatment issues. F-56

Have the patient identify her preferred music by selecting the music to be played, and then stating why she prefers the music. F-32

Assess the patient's music preferences by asking the patient to sing a cappella a song of her choice. Follow by playing on the piano the song that the patient sang, in the key in which it was sung. F-26

L-2 Demonstrates familiarity with and enjoyment of a variety of styles of music; respects the musical preferences of others; listens attentively to song and lyrics; focuses on the meaning of lyrics ($n^3 = 8$; $n^4 = 8$; $n^5 = 16$; 14.29%)

After playing a song, have the patient state what the song is about, how it relates to his or herself, the style of music, and whether or not he or she likes the song. M-30; M-51; F-30-32-35-51

Ask the patient to listen to a song then select one line related to current issues. M-41; F-41

Encourage each patient to listen to, and to make supportive statements regarding the musical preferences of other group members. M-26; F-26

Observe whether the patient participates in lyric analysis. M-40

Ask the patient to bring a song to the music therapy session that describes a topic of interest. M-85

Given a style of music, have the patient choose a song representative of the style. M-75

Observe the patient's willingness to listen to different styles of music and to participate in group discussions about contrasting styles. F-41

Have a group discussion in which each patient tells the group his favorite songs and performers, then plays a recording of the song for the group. M-31

Observe whether the patient refrains from speaking while listening to music. F-25

L-3   Shares personal knowledge or recollections associated with musical preferences; contributes to group discussions about music; demonstrates the ability to recognize and relate specific musical qualities or characteristics to personal preferences and significant life memories; relates abstract concepts in music to one's own experience ($n^3 = 6$; $n^4 = 3$; $n^5 = 9$; 8.04%)

Ask the patient to listen to a song and, based upon the patient's familiarity with the song, share information, ideas, or memories relating to the song lyrics or music. M-41-30; F-41

Ask the patient to request or identify some favorite songs. After listening to each song, ask the patient to explain the song's qualities and the particular personal significance of the song. M-40

Ask the patient to listen to a song while thinking of memories, ideas, hopes, wishes, and feelings he would like to keep. Draw a picture of a bottle and ask the patient to imagine the bottle signifies himself. Tell the patient you are going to play the song, "Time in a Bottle." Ask the patient to list, while the song is playing, memories or things he would like to keep inside the bottle. Also, the patient should list, or put outside the bottle, things he would like to forget, or get rid of. M-35

During lyric analysis, observe whether the patient is able to relate personal issues (e.g., his home life) to the song lyrics. After listening to the song, prompt the patient to discuss his family life and his future goals. M-31

Present the patient with a variety of songs. Ask the patient to pick out one song that best describes herself, her day, and her future. Next, ask the patient to tell how or why the song describes herself, her day, and her future. F-20

Ask the patient to choose a song that describes her feelings and then to play the song for the group. F-26

Play a recording of a well-known performer and ask the group if they know anything about the performer or the song. Observe which patients contribute to the group discussion about the performer or the song. M-40

L-4 Chooses music to promote own relaxation; enjoys easy listening music ($n^3 = 1$; $n^4 = 5$; $n^5 = 6$; 5.36%)

Assess the patient's ability to use music listening to promote relaxation. Ask the patient to choose music for relaxation. Does the patient have sufficient attention span to participate in relaxation to music? Test the patient's ability to attend to a task for increasing periods of time (e.g., 10 minutes, then 15 minutes, etc.). M-30; F-30-60

Play ten relaxing music selections for the patient. Ask the patient to rate each selection in terms of how relaxing she perceives the music to be. F-35

Assess/develop the patient's ability to use both vocal and instrumental music to promote relaxation exercises. Have the patient do muscle relaxation exercises (tensing followed by relaxation of specific muscle groups) to instrumental music, and deep breathing to produce vocal tones. F-35

Play easy listening music and ask the patient to listen and describe any images that come to mind. F-30

L-5 Selects preferred music that expresses present or past feelings ($n^3 = 3$; $n^4 = 2$; $n^5 = 5$; 4.46%)

Present the patient with numerous recordings representing a variety of styles of music. Ask the patient to select a musical preference that expresses how he or she is feeling today or has felt in the past. M-41-26; F-41

Given a list of 300 songs, ask the patient to choose a song that describes how she feels, or which describes an issue she is presently working on. Encourage the patient to not choose her favorite song. F-56

After playing the music have patients talk about feelings they associate with the music. M-35

L-6 Demonstrates musical awareness when listening; exhibits discriminatory listening skills ($n^3 = 3$; $n^4 = 1$; $n^5 = 4$; 3.57%)

Ask the patient to complete a music listening questionnaire while listening to the music. Questions on the questionnaire should be focused toward assessing the patient's degree of musical awareness, and be arranged in order of difficulty from easy to difficult. Such questions, for example, might require the patient to identify the music played (e.g., composer, title, artist), identify the category or style of music, identify the instruments heard and any changing tempos, identify feelings elicited by the music, and rate the music on a scale of 1 to 10, with 1 being most preferred. Patient may be asked to give an explanation of their rating. M-75; F-30

Play a variety of styles of music and ask the patients to identify the style being played. M-35

Teach the patients to hear chord changes while listening to recorded music. M-30

L-7 Demonstrates the ability to associate affect with corresponding music; verbalizes perceived mood of preferred music; identifies the mood of the music ($n^3 = 1$; $n^4 = 3$; $n^5 = 4$; 3.57%)

The patient listens to preferred music she has previously selected and verbalizes her perceptions of the mood of the music. F-32

Give the patient two musical selections with an explanation of the nature of the pieces if they are unfamiliar. After listening to the selections ask the patient to express his opinion of the selections. M-40

Play unfamiliar instrumental music compositions that have descriptive song titles (e.g., "Listen to the Wind," "Dance of the Windup Toy," "Rain"). Have the patients guess the song title, or to make up a title to the music. F-32

Play "The Erlking" (Schubert, 1815). Ask patients to identify feelings they perceive in the music. NOTE: "The Erlking" ("Der Erlkonig") is a song about "...the tragic ride of a father trying to out distance the Erlking, Death. The three characters of Goethe's poem are portrayed in the voice part: the child who sees Death, the father who tries to give him courage, and the enticing voice of the Erlking. Suggesting rapid hoof beats and a pounding pulse, the piano accompaniment keeps an exciting rhythm going throughout. Only at the end, on a dark chord, the Neapolitan sixth, ...does the motion stop. The singer gasps the final line, 'In his arms the child was dead,' and the song is over (Lloyd, 1968, p. 513)." F-30

L-8 Recognizes or recalls the titles of well-known, age-appropriate songs when they are played ($n^3 = 0$; $n^4 = 3$; $n^5 = 3$; 2.68%)

Conduct the "Name That Tune" activity to assist patients in identifying the melody of familiar songs. Use songs that have been played in previous music therapy sessions. The songs presented should have recovery themes. If patients have difficulty identifying the name of the song, provide cues or prompts (e.g., Play the song, "The Rose." If the patients do not respond ask them to name some songs with the word "rose" in the title). F-60; F-30

Conduct a "Name That Tune" activity. Play songs and ask residents to name their titles. F-25

L-9 Chooses a song for group listening ($n^3 = 2$; $n^4 = 1$; $n^5 = 3$; 2.68%)

The patient is give a list of 100 songs from which to choose. If the patient's favorite song is not on the list, ask the patient to name a song to add to the list. After singing the song the therapists may wish to involve the patients in a discussion of the lyrics. M-40; F-50

If the patient enjoys playing recordings for the group, arrange for the patient to serve as the disc jockey at the next patient party. M-25

L-10 Distinguishes and identifies characteristics of music (e.g., dynamics, tempo, timbre) ($n^3 = 2$; $n^4 = 1$; $n^5 = 3$; 2.68%)

Have the patient match the changes in the music by playing a rhythm instrument (e.g., plays loud to loud music, slow to slow music). M-30; F-30

Assess the resident's ability to distinguish between instruments of different timbre. Ask the resident to close his eyes. Play two different instrumental timbres (e.g., the drum followed by a resonator bell). Ask the resident to identify whether the timbres were the same or different. Next ask the resident to identify the name of the instruments played and the order in which they were played. M-25

L-11 Listens to music but does not identify musical preferences; may fear peers will not like choice of music ($n^3 = 1$; $n^4 = 2$; $n^5 = 3$; 2.68%)

Play various styles of music and ask the patient to listen to the music and rate his or her preference for it. M-51; F-51

Ask the patient to play her favorite recording, then to ask her peers what the song makes them think of. F-20

L-12 Chooses music that describes self ($n^3 = 1$; $n^4 = 2$; $n^5 = 3$; 2.68%)

Give the patient numerous recordings and ask him to choose a song that describes himself. M-35

Ask the patient to introduce herself to the group by picking a song that best describes herself. F-60

Given her preferred song, ask the patient to choose a sentence from the song that best describes herself. F-39

L-13 Identifies the names of musical instruments used in a recording ($n^3 = 2$; $n^4 = 0$; $n^5 = 2$; 1.79%)

Ask the patient to listening to a recording and to identify the names of any music instruments recognized. M-32

Play a music recording in which the sounds of specific instruments can be heard. Associate the sound of an instrument with the actual instrument, or a picture of the instrument. Follow by fading out visual aids so the patient can identify the instrument from an aural presentation. M-31

L-14 Demonstrates the ability to perceive music ($n^3 = 1$; $n^4 = 1$; $n^5 = 2$; 1.79%)

Ask the patient to demonstrate an observable response to the music as it is playing (i.e., facial, movement). M-30

During music listening, observe any unprompted physical responses to the beat or rhythm. F-30

L-15   Sleeps when listening to music (apparently enjoys music listening as evidenced by regular attendance to the listening laboratory) ($n^3 = 1$; $n^4 = 1$; $n^5 = 2$; 1.79%)

Provide the patient with colored pencils and paper. Ask the patient to draw his or her impressions while listening to the music. M-21; F-21

L-16   Patient listens to one recording repeatedly, in multiple succession to the exclusion of other recordings ($n^3 = 1$; $n^4 = 1$; $n^5 = 2$; 1.79%)

Provide positive reinforcement (e.g., tokens, points, or edibles) for choosing to listen to different music. M-21; F-21

L-17   Demonstrates knowledge of relaxing music ($n^3 = 1$; $n^4 = 1$; $n^5 = 2$; 1.79%)

The patient is given a list of relaxing musical recordings and asked to choose her preferred recordings for future listening. M-51; F-51

L-18   Uses musical equipment independently ($n^3 = 0$; $n^4 = 1$; $n^5 = 1$; 00.89%)

Ask the patient to use a variety of music listening equipment (e.g., tape recorder, record player, video tape player, compact disc player) then observe her ability to use it. F-30

L-19   Listens to music independently ($n^3 = 0$; $n^4 = 1$; $n^5 = 1$; 00.89%)

Observe whether the patient listens to music during her leisure time. F-30

L-20   Demonstrates the ability to locate sound sources ($n^3 = 1$; $n^4 = 0$; $n^5 = 1$; 00.89%)

Ask the patient to close his eyes. The therapist turns on a sound source located in the room, then asks the patient to open his eyes and to point to where the music is coming from. M-25

L-21   Chooses music that describes a peer ($n^3 = 0$; $n^4 = 1$; $n^5 = 1$; 00.89%)

During group listening, give a patient numerous recordings and ask her to choose a song that describes personal qualities of the peer on her left. F-60

L-22   Prefers specific elements of music ($n^3 = 0$; $n^4 = 1$; $n^5 = 1$; 00.89%)

Play a preferred song for the patient. Ask the patient whether they prefer the lyrics, the melody, or the beat of the song best. F-31

L-23 Expresses likes as well as dislikes regarding a musical selection ($n^3 = 0$; $n^4 = 1$; $n^5 = 1$; 00.89%)

Select a variety of songs representative of the style of music the patient prefers. Each song selected should be different from the others, in terms of tempo, volume, orchestration, and the theme of the lyrics. Play the songs and ask the patient to indicate their relative preference for the songs by rating the songs on a five point scale. After the patient finishes rating the songs, assist the patient in making decisions about what she specifically likes or dislikes about each song. Also, ask the patient to identify professional performing groups that sound similar to her preferred songs. F-31

L-24 Chooses appropriate background music ($n^3 = 0$; $n^4 = 1$; $n^5 = 1$; 00.89%)

During a poetry writing session, assign a patient to choose appropriate background music to play during the recitation of the poem. The music should be appropriate to the mood and content of the poem. F-31

SINGING
(Combined, n = 75; 20.60%; Male, $n^1 = 28$; 37.33%; Female, $n^2 = 47$; 62.67%)

BEHAVIOR

S-1 Participates in group sing-a-long; sings with group to piano or guitar accompaniment; indicates a desire to sing ($n^3 = 7$; $n^4 = 9$; $n^5 = 16$; 21.33%)

MUSIC THERAPY INTERVENTION

Observe quality of participation (e.g., cooperates, takes turns requesting songs, sings in harmony with others, rhythm, vocal tone; pitch). M-30-25; F-37-30-65

Have the patients make decisions about which songs to sing during an informal sing-a-long. Given a list of 30 songs, have each patient select one song for the group to sing. M-25-35; F-26-32

Ask the patient to select a song from a song list for the group to sing, and then to sing the song with the group. M-32-30; F-35

Give patients the opportunity to sing Blues songs.

Ask the patient to name any song for the group to sing, such as their favorite or most memorable song. F-30

Encourage patients to talk about their favorite groups during the sing-a-long. Use the patients' preferred music in the sing-a-long. If a patient is experienced at playing piano, guitar, or drums, invite the patient to use their instrument to accompany the sing-a-long. M-25

Give the patient a music instrument and ask the patient to play the instrument while singing (order this task according to the ability level of the patient). F-41

Allot time for song dedication during the sing-a-long. Ask each patient to select a song and dedicate it to a peer. The group then sings the song. F-60

S-2 Performs a vocal solo before the group; expresses a desire to perform a vocal solo, or to perform on stage; spontaneously sings a solo ($n^3 = 3$; $n^4 = 9$; $n^5 = 12$; 16%)

Arrange for the patient to sing a solo before an audience (e.g., at the weekly talent show; ask the patient to select a favorite song from a booklet of patriotic songs to sing at the Fourth of July unit picnic). F-25-30-35

The patient rehearses with the therapist a song of choice to sing for the group. M-25

Identify the name of the song the patient most often sings before her peers. Praise the patient for singing a solo. During the group sing-a-long, ask the patient to sing each verse solo and the group to join in on the chorus. An alternative is to have the patient sing each chorus solo and the group to join in on the verse. F-30

Ask the patient to choose a song, then to sing the song through a microphone during the weekly sing-a-long. F-35

During the talent show, ask the patient to select any song (not limited to the song book) and to sing the song for the group using a microphone. F-35

Have the patient select a song, practice the song, then perform a vocal solo of the song before an audience (e.g., the Christmas pageant). F-30

The patient will sing at least 50% of a song, with no prompts, in front of a group of familiar people. M-30

Arrange a room with stage lights and chairs. Have the patient give a recital in which he sings his favorite songs. M-31

Ask the patient to pick a song that will "help her make it through the day." Arrange for the patient to sing the song to the group to reinforce the positive benefit of the song lyrics, and to boost the patient's self-esteem. F-30

Do a group rap that requires each patient to chant a solo line. F-65

S-3 Sings and follows a choral part ($n^3 = 3$; $n^4 = 2$; $n^5 = 5$; 6.67%)

Demonstrate to the patient how to sing and follow a choral part. Encourage the patient to ask for assistance if needed. M-30; F-30

Observe the patient's ability to harmonize and blend own voice with the group. M-25; F-32

Observe the patient's ability to read music notation. If unable to read music notation, observe the patient's ability to sing familiar songs from song lyrics. Teach the melody by rote to patients who cannot match the melody to the lyrics. M-31

S-4 Participates in a choir ($n^3 = 1$; $n^4 = 4$; $n^5 = 5$; 6.67%)

Assign the patients to a choir. During choir rehearsal work on social skills, cooperation, listening to and following directions, singing correct parts in harmonization with the chorus, and voice blending and balancing. To provide a goal for the choir to work toward, arrange for the choir to perform four concerts per year. M-75; F-26-32

During warm-up activities work on patients blending their voices with the group. F-32

When Christmas approaches, arrange for the patients to go caroling from ward to ward with a hospital wide group. Observe the patient's ability to function in moderate to large groups. F-30

S-5 Completes music questionnaire. Past singing performance is assessed by administering a music experience questionnaire ($n^3 = 2$; $n^4 = 2$; $n^5 = 4$; 5.33%).

If the patient indicates a strong preference for singing, ask the patient to request a favorite song, then accompany as the patient sings the song. Observe vocal skill, lyric accuracy, and awareness of style and composer. M-26; F-50

If the patient indicates experience at singing in the church choir, play a patient-familiar church song (e.g., "Amazing Grace"). Observe the patient's vocal skills, such as awareness of key or the ability to sing in key. M-26

If the patient indicates a desire to learn songs, to sing, or to harmonize, provide group or individual voice lessons. F-50

S-6 Exhibits superior vocal skill ($n^3 = 1$; $n^4 = 2$; $n^5 = 3$; 4%)

Patients who possess good vocal skill are good candidates for high status roles such as leading group singing. M-21; F-21

Enroll in voice lessons and expand knowledge of musical concepts and styles. F-36

S-7 Sings only one style of music (e.g., gospel, rock, or country, etc.) ($n^3 = 1$; $n^4 = 2$; $n^5 = 3$; 4%)

Although the patient desires to learn other types of music, he or she doesn't because of continuously singing, for example, gospel. Make the singing of one gospel song at the end of the session contingent upon singing a variety of styles of music during the music therapy session. To promote generalization, give the patient a checklist with various styles of music. Have the patient keep the checklist, checking the style of music each time he or she sings a song outside the music therapy session. Emphasize the necessity of singing a variety of styles, and ask the patient to bring the checklist to the next music therapy session for review. M-21; F-21

Involve the patient in a sing-a-long group to increase exposure to a variety of styles of music. F-36

S-8   Demonstrates vocal range ($n^3 = 1$; $n^4 = 2$; $n^5 = 3$; 4%)

Begin choir with vocal warm-ups. During warm-ups work at increasing vocal range. Increased vocal range will lead to increased confidence in singing activities. M-30; F-31

Do five-note ascending-descending vocal warm-up exercises starting on middle "C" and continuing through "G^1." Follow by singing a song in the range of the vocal warm-ups. F-31

S-9   Sings at least two lines of a song from memory ($n^3 = 1$; $n^4 = 2$; $n^5 = 3$; 4%)

Ask the patient to select a familiar song and to sing as much of the song as possible. NOTE: Transpose the song to the patient's vocal range. M-41; F-25-41

S-10   Sings with correct pitch and rhythm ($n^3 = 2$; $n^4 = 0$; $n^5 = 2$; 2.67%)

Observe the ability of the patient to sing on pitch (The patient chooses the song and the therapist accompanies on guitar or piano). M-30-40

S-11   Matches pitch ($n^3 = 1$; $n^4 = 1$; $n^5 = 2$; 2.67%)

Observe whether the patient first listens to the pitch before attempting to match it. Model correct listening-matching response. Encourage the patient to practice listening before matching. M-30; F-30

S-12   Sings with appropriate dynamics ($n^3 = 1$; $n^4 = 1$; $n^5 = 2$; 2.67%)

Teach the patients to blend vocally with others. Encourage the patients to listen to themselves, to each other, and to watch and sing according to the conductor's cues. M-30; F-31

S-13   The patient requests voice lessons; expresses a desire to sing a solo of a favorite song ($n^3 = 1$; $n^4 = 1$; $n^5 = 2$; 2.67%)

During voice lessons stress proper breathing, posture, and diction. M-75

Work on deep breathing, vocalization, song interpretation, and posture. Involve the patient in a discussion of the lyrics. Encourage the patient to sing with others in addition to singing solo. F-37

S-14 Demonstrates the ability to use the voice expressively; feels comfortable expressing oneself in song ($n^3 = 1$; $n^4 = 1$; $n^5 = 2$; 2.67%)

Encourage the patient to use both body movement and vocal sounds to express a particular mood or emotion. M-40

Ask the patient to pick a song to sing that she feels describes herself. F-20

S-15 Stays on task during singing activities; Indicates preference for singing ($n^3 = 0$; $n^4 = 2$; $n^5 = 2$; 2.67%)

Give directives and ask questions to maintain on-task behavior (e.g., Ask the patient to pick a song and then to sing the song. Ask the patient questions relating to the song). F-20

Observe the patients on-task behavior during a sing-a-long (e.g., attention to song). F-60

S-16 Sings with breath control and appropriate intensity ($n^3 = 0$; $n^4 = 1$; $n^5 = 1$; 1.33%)

Start by singing the chorus and one verse of a song (e.g., "Amazing Grace"). After a short break have the patient sing the chorus and another verse. Gradually increase the length of time singing without a break. F-31

S-17 Participates in toning exercises; demonstrates the ability to sing (match) the intonation sung by the leader of the toning activity ($n^3 = 0$; $n^4 = 1$; $n^5 = 1$; 1.33%)

During toning exercises the group is instructed to follow the toning exercises of the leader. Each group member is given the opportunity to be the leader and to change the toning pattern. F-60

S-18 Sings both a cappella and with accompaniment ($n^3 = 1$; $n^4 = 0$; $n^5 = 1$; 1.33%)

Ask the patient to sing a few bars of his favorite melody, after which the therapist joins in with an instrumental accompaniment (if possible). M-40

S-19 Demonstrates physiological aspects of vocalization ($n^3 = 0$; $n^4 = 1$; $n^5 = 1$; 1.33%)

Observe quality of deep breathing, vocalization, or any need for speech correction. M-35

S-20 Sings lyrics to an entire song ($n3 = 0$; $n^4 = 1$; $n^5 = 1$; 1.33%)

Provide a piano accompaniment to a familiar song (e.g.," America") and encourage the residents to sing along. Note whether the residents can sing the words to the entire song. NOTE: Transpose the song to the patient's vocal range. F-25

S-21 Sings lyrics to only phrases of songs ($n^3 = 0$; $n^4 = 1$; $n^5 = 1$; 1.33%)

The therapist sings and plays the first half of the first phrase of a familiar song (e.g., "America"). Observe whether the resident can sing the lyrics to the remainder of the phrase while the therapist accompanies. NOTE: Transpose the song to the patient's vocal range. F-25

S-22 Sings song lyrics in sequence ($n^3 = 0$; $n^4 = 1$; $n^5 = 1$; 1.33%)

Ask the patient to sing a familiar song, or to sing one line of a familiar song. Observe whether the lyrics are sung in the correct sequence. F-25

S-23 Performance anxiety; experiences anxiety about singing for others ($n^3 = 1$; $n^4 = 0$; $n^5 = 1$; 1.33%)

Have the patient participate in a choir and schedule a concert every two to three months. Process performance anxiety feelings about each concert both before and after the concert. M-30

S-24 Expresses likes and dislikes about a song, or portions of the song ($n^3 = 0$; $n^4 = 1$; $n^5 = 1$; 1.33%)

After singing songs discuss the songs with the patient. Note whether the patient expresses both likes and dislikes about songs. F-35

PLAYING INSTRUMENTS
(Combined, $n = 65$; 17.86%; Male, $n^1 = 30$; 46.15%; Female, $n^2 = 35$; 53.85%)

BEHAVIOR

P-1 Demonstrates musical interest; may spontaneously play or attempt to play a musical instrument; may or may not exhibit instrumental skill ($n^3 = 11$; $n^4 = 21$; $n^5 = 32$; 49.23%)

MUSIC THERAPY INTERVENTION

Increase the patient's musical skill. Help the patient learn or relearn a musical skill. Provide regularly scheduled lessons on the patient's instrument of choice (e.g., voice, piano, guitar, autoharp) in a group or one-to-one session. Encourage daily practice. Increase peer acceptance, self-esteem, and confidence by preparing the patient to perform for her peers (e.g., on the patient variety or talent show or at a ward birthday party). Involve the patient in a combo to promote small group interaction and peer acceptance. Encourage the patient to continue using her musical skills after leaving the hospital. Suggest community involvement in music after discharge from the hospital. Consider giving the patient the opportunity to continue taking lessons from the therapist through direct or community referral after release from the hospital. Prepare to focus on primary psychotherapeutic (nonmusic) goals. M-21-30-30; F-21-30-30-30-31-31-35-36-37-50-60

Provide the patient with a variety of musical instruments such as piano, guitar, drums, autoharp, and xylophone. Assess the patient's ability to play an instrument and to read music. M-40; F-36-30

Patients who demonstrate advanced performance ability on guitar or piano may be auditioned for a coveted role, such as providing background music for an exercise group. Giving a music performance can be a means of self expression, or of gaining peer acceptance. M-21; F-21-39

Observe whether the patient plays an instrument well enough to derive personal satisfaction and enjoyment from playing. M-30-60

If the patient wishes to learn the drum part of a recording, assist the patient with listening analytically to that part of the recording. M-51; F-51

Give the patient the opportunity to engage in solo experimentation on preferred instruments (e.g., piano, drum). M-30; F-39

Involve the patient in a band in which she can perform written as well as improvised music. F-20

Assess the patient's present guitar playing ability by asking the patient if he plays guitar. If he indicates he does, give him a guitar and ask him to play it. If the patient possesses at least minimal functional guitar skill, encourage him to play the guitar during his free time while in the hospital. Give the patient the opportunity to check out the guitar, for use during his free time, by signing the "sign-out" or "instrument use" book. Monitor the sign-out book to determine whether the patient regularly checks out the guitar. M-40

Encourage the patient to practice several songs they enjoy, then invite several peers or staff to come and listen to the patient. M-31

Ask the patient to practice with the therapist at least one hour twice a week. F-25

Ask the patient to identify the style of music she wishes to perform, and specific songs representative of the style. F-32

After performing selected music, the patient will evaluate her performance by identifying aspects of the music that was performed well and performed inaccurately. F-32

P-2 **Demonstrates sufficient ability to perform solo or with an ensemble; maintains tempo and rhythm; plays dynamics ($n^3 = 5$; $n^4 = 4$; $n^5 = 9$; 13.85%)**

Observe the patient's ability to perform with a group. Does the patient use appropriate dynamic levels and tempo when performing with others? Does the patient perform as a contributing member? M-30-85; F-60

Ask the patient to play a prearranged accompaniment on Orff instruments as the therapist plays a pentatonic song incorporating two to three chords. Provide the patient with different prearranged accompaniments for different Orff instruments. Observe the patient's ability to stay in tempo with the pentatonic song. M-35-35; F-32

Ask the patient to keep time to recorded music using their preferred rhythm instrument. Observe the patient's ability to play rhythm instruments in time with the group. F-30; F-26

For the patient who wishes to perform (play the drums) but has difficulty keeping a steady tempo, ask the patient to play along with a radio or recording. Encourage the patient to keep a steady beat. This activity helps to increase the person's self confidence that they can maintain a steady beat. M-31.

P-3 | Performance anxiety; expresses desire to play for others but is fearful of solo playing; may be quiet and passive ($n^3 = 2$; $n^4 = 4$; $n^5 = 6$; 9.23%)

Accompany the patient's performance. If the patient wishes to play, for example, a guitar solo during group sing-a-long, the therapist should accompany the patient's performance using a second guitar. M-51; F-51

During the patient's music lesson, have the patient play for one or two peers. During combo rehearsal, have the patient play his or her instrument before the other group members. Have regularly scheduled combo concerts to enable the patient to play for progressively larger audiences. Process performance anxiety feelings about each concert both before and after the concert. M-30; F-20

Arrange for the patient to play for the music therapist at least twice a week. F-31

Observe the patient's willingness to play an instrument during group instrumental activities or to participate in a talent show or play. F-41

P-4 | Performs in group ensemble for peers; expresses a desire to perform with the hospital performance group. ($n^3 = 4$; $n^4 = 1$; $n^5 = 5$; 7.69%)

Involve the patients in an instrumental performance ensemble (e.g., hand bells; guitar). Have the group perform for facility and community functions. Emphasize group process. M-75-30

Involve the patient in a group ensemble. Let the group take the responsibility for choosing the music and making all arrangements for the concert, which is to be given for their peers. If desired, arrangements may be made for certain patients to perform a vocal or instrumental solo during the concert. M-25

During combo rehearsal, teach the patients to hear chord changes by listening to recorded music. After identifying the chord changes, have them transcribe the music into lead sheet format. M-30

For patients who wish to learn piano, begin by teaching the patient to identify piano note names. Next teach right and left hand placements for playing simple I, IV, and V block chord progressions in various keys. F-31

P-5 Assess past instrumental performance by administering a music experience questionnaire (n^3 = 3; n^4 = 1; n^5 = 4; 6.15%).

Patient indicates any instrumental or vocal experience. M-30; F-30

If the patient indicates experience at playing the guitar, give him a guitar and ask him to pluck the "D" string. M-26

If the patient indicates he can read music, present him with music symbols and ask him to name the symbols (e.g., treble clef, quarter note, common [4/4] time signature). M-26

P-6 Demonstrates the ability to imitate or repeat a rhythmic or melodic phrase (n^3 = 2; n^4 = 1; n^5 = 3; 4.62%)

For rhythmic imitation, play a rhythmic pattern on a drum and ask the patient to repeat the pattern. For melodic imitation, play a melodic pattern on an Orff instrument and ask the patient to repeat the pattern. M-35-35; F-32

P-7 Patient expresses a desire accompany own singing (n^3 = 1; n^4 = 1; n^5 = 2; 3.08%)

For patients with little instrumental skill, provide autoharp or omnichord instruction. M-51; F-51

P-8 Plays predetermined pattern on tone bells to create a familiar song (n^3 = 1; n^4 = 1; n^5 = 2; 3.08%)

Given a musical reference, ask the patient to play the melody of a familiar song on tone bells. Determine whether the patient reads notation, note letter names, or numbers. M-30; F-30

P-9 Participates in informal "jam session" (n^3 = 1; n^4 = 0; n^5 = 1; 1.54%)

Have the patients attend sessions that allow them to interact with other patients having varied levels of music skill. Encourage participants to learn songs from each other as well as teach songs. The level of participation can be as simple as playing a rhythm instrument or as complex as playing the guitar, drums, piano, or a wind instrument. M-75

P-10 Performs a variety of musical styles; demonstrates tolerance for the music preferences of others (n^3 = 0; n^4 = 1; n^5 = 1; 1.54%)

Alternate patient-preferred music with other styles of music. Ask the patients to identify different elements of the music, such as the melody, bass, and percussion. F-31

IMPROVISING MUSIC
(Combined, n = 54; 14.83%; Male, n^1 = 22; 40.74%; Female, n^2 = 32; 59.26%)

BEHAVIOR

I-1 Plays Orff and rhythm instruments during free or structured improvisation sessions (n^3 = 6; n^4 = 12; n^5 = 18; 33.33%)

MUSIC THERAPY INTERVENTION

Observe the patient's quality of participation in group improvisation (e.g., trades instruments with peers upon request; follows auditory cues by ceasing to play instrument when accompaniment or leader stops playing; cooperates and follows directions; plays at appropriate times; demonstrates creativity; listens to others and plays as a group member rather than as an individual; works with group to create finished product). Observe whether each patient improvises a pattern, or contributes a song or song line, a thought, a word, or an idea to be depicted. M-25-41; F-25-35-39-41-65

Ask the patient to use percussion accessories to provide an improvisation to a recording. M-51; F-37-51

Observe the patient's instrumental facility (e.g., the number of instruments the patient is able to play and the quality of improvisation). M-25; F-65

Observe the patient's quality of free improvisation on Orff and rhythm instruments. Does the patient demonstrate flexibility and creativity? Is the patient able to be creative while experimenting with rhythm and tone? F-30-39

Ask the patient to choose two or three chord progressions on which to base a guitar improvisation. M-32

Given a harmonic structure as an accompaniment, the patient is able to improvise at least a 12-bar melody on her preferred melodic instrument. F-35

Given instrument of choice, ask the patient to choose an ostinato pattern on which to perform with the group. M-32

During structured improvisation, encourage the resident to improvise on an instrument to an underlying ostinato (e.g., one patient or the group plays the ostinato while another resident plays an improvisation). F-25

I-2 Expresses feelings and expressiveness through music improvisation; demonstrates the ability to play the sound of a feeling. (n^3 = 3; n^4 = 4; n^5 = 7; 12.96%)

Observe whether the patient can convey emotional responses through a sound medium. Ask the patient to play an instrument in a manner that expresses his or her mood. After the patient finishes playing, ask the patient to verbalize his or her mood. M-30; F-60

Ask the patient to choose an instrument that matches a mood or a day she has experienced (e.g., "Choose an instrument that reminds you of _____.").

Ask the patient to play the instrument. Discuss with the patient how she felt when playing, and if it was a sound she could modify. F-31

Ask the patient to select an instrument of choice, then communicate his current affect or feeling by expressively playing the instrument. M-40

Have the patient express feelings by using instruments to create original sound effects and to match specific emotions. M-35

Give the patient a card with a specific feeling written on it. Ask the patient to play the sound of the feeling on a rhythm instrument. F-60

Using the pentatonic scale and Orff instruments, assign a patient to improvise appropriate background music during the recitation of a poem. The music should be appropriate to the mood and content of the poem. F-39

I-3 Maintains ostinato pattern; plays rhythmically; keeps a steady beat ($n^3 = 3$; $n^4 = 2$; $n^5 = 5$; 9.26%)

Play a one or two measure rhythmic pattern on a drum and observe the patient's ability to imitate the pattern. M-25

The patient chooses an ostinato pattern and establishes the tempo. F-32

The therapist plays "La Bamba" on the guitar or piano while the patient creates a rhythmic accompaniment to the music using the claves. The therapist also may assign the patient to play a set, or structured rhythmic accompaniment throughout the song (e.g., $\mathbf{C}$ | || | |). M-26

Using a rhythm instrument activity, the leader plays an ostinato rhythmic pattern on a drum. The group members join in one by one, each imitating the leader's rhythmic pattern on their instrument. M-35; F-32

I-4 Improvises a rhythm or melody over a rhythmic or melodic ostinato pattern ($n^3 = 1$; $n^4 = 4$; $n^5 = 5$; 9.26%)

Using Orff instruments, present a rhythmic and/or melodic ostinato pattern and ask the patient to improvise a melody over the pattern. M-35; F-32-35

Teach the patient a melodic pattern on her preferred instrument. F-32

Observe the patient's ability to play a counter beat, an alternating beat, and her own rhythmic pattern in the presence of a steady beat played by the therapist. F-35

I-5 Feels musically inferior; the patient is convinced she cannot play music; exhibits excessive fear of musical failure and fear of musical participation; exhibits low self-confidence and low self-esteem; makes negative statements such as "I can't" ($n^3 = 2$; $n^4 = 2$; $n^5 = 4$; 7.41%)

Use improvisational techniques to provide the patient with positive and successful musical experiences (e.g., prepare the patient to perform an ostinato part). M-40; F-50

Involve the patient in structured improvisation. M-40

Use nontraditional instrumental techniques and/or the pentatonic scale to facilitate success (e.g., Set the electronic piano or keyboard to play a rhythmic accompaniment. Using the pentatonic scale, have the patient improvise a melody to the rhythmic accompaniment by playing the black keys on the keyboard or by playing a melodic percussion instrument such as the xylophone). Encourage peer acceptance and praise of the performance. F-30

I-6   Demonstrates preference for improvisational instruments ($n^3 = 1$; $n^4 = 2$; $n^5 = 3$; 5.56%)

Given improvisational instruments for ensemble playing, each patient will choose her preferred instrument. M-41; F-32-41

I-7   Demonstrates the ability to musically imitate, alternate, and initiate during improvisation ($n^3 = 2$; $n^4 = 1$; $n^5 = 3$; 5.56%)

Observe whether the patient initiates verbal or nonverbal participation with the therapist or a peer. Using rhythm instruments, try a mirroring to music activity in which the therapist or a peer leads and the patient follows. Repeat the activity with the patient leading and the therapist or peer following. NOTE: A two measure improvised rhythm pattern is suggested. Observe how many times the leader must present the rhythm pattern before the patient can correctly repeat or echo the pattern. M-25; F-30

Ask the patient to engage in musical mirroring, followed by musical conversation with the therapist. M-40

I-8   The patient expresses a desire to improvise at the piano ($n^3 = 1$; $n^4 = 2$; $n^5 = 3$; 5.56%)

For patients with little piano background, involve the patient in a pentatonic duet (the therapist improvises on the black keys in one register of the keyboard while the patient improvises on the black keys in another register). M-51; F-51

Provide experience at unstructured, guided improvisation. Have the residents play a pentatonic improvisation on the black keys of the piano. Suggest a scene (e.g., a thunderstorm) for the residents to create or represent through their improvisation. F-25

I-9   Expresses creativity during group improvisation; creatively explores instrument ($n^3 = 1$; $n^4 = 1$; $n^5 = 2$; 3.70%)

The patient will improvise at least two varied rhythms, without prompts, while playing the hand drum during group improvisation. M-30

Ask the patient to nonverbally "say something" while playing the xylophone to the therapist's accompaniment. The patient may use only xylophone playing and nonverbal gestures to communicate. F-25

I-10 Feels at ease with playing a variety of sounds on different Orff instruments ($n^3 = 0$; $n^4 = 1$; $n^5 = 1$; 1.85%)

Teach the patient a simple ostinato pattern on her chosen instrument. After the patient learns the pattern, ask her to vary the sound while maintaining the same pattern. Repeat until the patient plays three different versions of the same pattern on a variety of Orff instruments. F-31

I-11 Leads or conducts group improvisation sessions ($n^3 = 0$; $n^4 = 1$; $n^5 = 1$; 1.85%)

Ask the patient to use the baton to indicate changes in musical characteristics such as dynamics and tempo. F-35

I-12 "Hears" chord changes ($n^3 = 1$; $n^4 = 0$; $n^5 = 1$; 1.85%)

The therapist provides the patient with a guitar so that both the therapist and the patient have a guitar. The patient and therapist then play their guitars while singing a familiar song. Observe whether the patient changes chords at the appropriate times (NOTE: The therapist may need to use nontraditional, simplified guitar techniques, or restrict the patient's role to providing a one-note accompaniment on the xylophone, bass keyboard, or guitar). M-26

I-13 Interacts with other group members while improvising ($n^3 = 1$; $n^4 = 0$; $n^5 = 1$; 1.85%)

Ask the patient to improvise a response to an improvised statement made by another group member. M-35

I-14 Improvises movements to music (see "Participates in unstructured creative movement to music" under "Locomotor Movement to Music")

LOCOMOTOR MOVEMENT TO MUSIC
(Combined, n = 31; 8.52%; Male, $n^1 = 8$; 25.81%; Female, $n^2 = 23$; 74.19%)

BEHAVIOR

LM-1 Dances to music (e.g., ballroom, square, folk); participates in structured dance; participates in dance mixer or social dance; may demonstrate previous dancing experience ($n^3 = 2$; $n^4 = 6$; $n^5 = 8$; 25.81%)

MUSIC THERAPY INTERVENTION

Play dance music and invite the patients to participate in dancing. Observe whether patients participate independently or with prompts. F-35-41

Ask the patient with prior dancing experience to assist the therapist in teaching a dance (e.g., a square dance) to the group. M-21; F-21

Play patient preferred music, or play "patient era" music if the musical preferences of the patient are unknown. Instrumental "dance era" music is recommended. THERAPIST NOTE: Ballroom dancing is the style of dance most preferred by my patients. M-40

Observe whether the patient asks a peer to dance during coed dance (socialization) activities. F-35

Observe whether participation in dance or movement activities reduces the patient's symptoms of tension. F-30

Observe the patient's quality of rhythmic movement while she is dancing. F-36

LM-2   Participates in structured creative movement to music; imitates or mirrors movements to music ($n^3 = 2$; $n^4 = 3$; $n^5 = 5$; 16.13%)

Ask the patients to imitate a leader in creative movement activities. The patients take turns being the leader, or the therapist can be the leader. M-25; F-25-26

Divide the patients into pairs. Ask the first patient of each pair to move to the music while the second patient imitates the movement. Follow by having the patients switch roles (i.e., the second patient assumes the first patient's role and the first patient assumes the second patient's role) so the imitation skills of all patients can be observed. M-25; F-65

LM-3   Participates in unstructured creative movement to music; spontaneously moves to music ($n^3 = 0$; $n^4 = 4$; $n^5 = 4$; 12.90%)

Assess the patient's spontaneous movement to music. Note any indications of psychiatric problems. F-26-37

Play music and encourage the residents to move independently to the music. Provide imagery for the residents to create and represent in their movements. Imagery, music, and movement may be used to energize the patients (e.g., Ask the patients to imitate African dance movements to the song, "The Rhythm Is Gonna Get You" by Miami Sound Machine). F-25

Ask the patients to select a movement that expresses something about themselves, and which will "pass" their energy. Observe their movements to previously selected recorded music. F-30

LM-4   Moves in rhythm to music ($n^3 = 1$; $n^4 = 2$; $n^5 = 3$; 9.68%)

Have the patient mirror the therapist's movements. Use appropriate prompting if necessary. M-25

Involve the patient in a music exercise or dance group in which the patient can learn basic movements or dance steps to music. F-20

Use structured movement exercise to rhythmic music with patients who have difficulty moving rhythmically or difficulty controlling voluntary movements. F-30

LM-5 Participates in aerobics ($n^3 = 0$; $n^4 = 3$; $n^5 = 3$; 9.68%)

Involve the patient in a music exercise group to increase physical movement, self-esteem, and self-image. F-20

Involve the patient in aerobic exercise to music. F-41

Involve the patient in choosing the music for dance aerobics and water aerobics. F-36

LM-6 Maintains the tempo of the music given directed gross motor movements ($n^3 = 1$; $n^4 = 1$; $n^5 = 2$; 6.45%)

Play a recording with a tempo of approximately 60 beats per minute and observe the patient's ability to do aerobic exercises in rhythm to the music. M-26; F-26

LM-7 Integrates and performs a structured movement pattern to music given verbal directives by the therapist ($n^3 = 1$; $n^4 = 1$; $n^5 = 2$; 6.45%)

Patient follows dance sequence to instrumental music. M-25

Design the movement pattern to serve the patient's physical and expressive needs. F-37

LM-8 Participates in creative dance and body language ($n^3 = 0$; $n^4 = 1$; $n^5 = 1$; 3.23%)

Involve the patient in a body language group to increase physical movement, self-esteem, and self-image. F-20

LM-9 Awareness of personal space or body limits during movement to music ($n^3 = 1$; $n^4 = 0$; $n^5 = 1$; 3.23%)

Observe whether the patient verbally identifies and physically responds to personal space limits (e.g., does not intrude upon the space of others; does not constantly bump into others). M-32

LM-10 Leads group in simple, repetitive creative movement ($n^3 = 0$; $n^4 = 1$; $n^5 = 1$; 3.23%)

Observe the patient leading the group in movement to music. F-32

LM-11 Feels comfortable with structured movement activity ($n^3 = 0$; $n^4 = 1$; $n^5 = 1$; 3.23%)

Use a game involving movement to music to assist patients in feeling comfortable with structured movement activities (e.g., Play the game, Who Started the Motion. This game involves structured movement to music. F-65

COMPOSING MUSIC

(Combined, n = 18; 4.95%; Male, n^1 = 7; 38.89%; Female, n^2 = 11; 61.11%)

BEHAVIOR

C-1 Patient participates in lyric writing; participates in setting lyrics to music (n^3 = 5; n^4 = 9; n^5 = 14; 77.78%)

MUSIC THERAPY INTERVENTION

The goal is to get a tangible "black and white" copy of the patient's true feelings. Does the patient write lyrics that reflect appropriate self awareness, emotion, and contact with the environment? Does the patient give suggestions for lyrics based on her own thoughts and feelings? M-35-30; F-39-60

During group song writing, give each group member a work sheet and ask each person to contribute to the parody. The melody used may be a familiar song (e.g., "Greatest Love of All"). F-60-65

Observe whether each patient contributes a line to the song, a thought, a word, or an idea to be depicted. F-39

Have each patient make up their own lyrical verse to the melody of a familiar song such as "Kum Bah Yah." F-26

During lyric writing, have each patient create one line of lyrics. F-31

Observe the quality of participation. Observe whether the patient communicates thoughts about lyrics and melody to the group, demonstrates creativity and flexibility, and works with the entire group in shaping the product. F-39

Involve the patient in writing lyrics in Blues form. The therapist uses a guitar to sing with the patient, lyrics already written, and to prompt the patient into thinking of and trying new lyrics. M-30

With the therapist's assistance, the patient decides which melody and chord progression best expresses the lyrics (which are reflective of the patient's feelings). M-35

Select a melody that is unknown to the patient then teach the patient to hum the melody. After the patient learns the melody ask the patient to compose lyrics to the melody. Give necessary assistance. M-35

Given a song (e.g., "I Am a Rock") with certain key lyrics deleted, have the patient to fill in the missing words (blanks) with words that describe herself. For example, in the chorus: "I am _____, I am _____." F-39

C-2 Patient expresses a desire to compose, sing or play own compositions (n^3 = 2; n^4 = 1; n^5 = 3; 16.67%)

Therapist provides coaching sessions with performance upon termination of sessions. M-21; F-21

During a one-to-one session, assist the patient at composing lyrics and music. Encourage a possible performance for peers and staff. M-31

C-3 Demonstrates the ability to learn a newly composed song by rote ($n^3 = 0$; $n^4 = 1$; $n^5 = 1$; 5.56%)

During group song writing, the patients learn to sing each phrase of the newly completed song by rote (e.g., the therapist sings a phrase, followed by the patients singing the same phrase in imitation of the therapist). F-60

NONLOCOMOTOR MOVEMENT TO MUSIC
(Combined, n = 9; 2.47%; Male, $n^1 = 5$; 55.56%; Female, $n^2 = 4$; 44.45%)

BEHAVIOR

NL-1 Imitates movements to music ($n^3 = 2$; $n^4 = 1$; $n^5 = 3$; 33.33%)

MUSIC THERAPY INTERVENTION

Use scarves to create a mirroring experience for patients. Divide the patients into pairs and give each patient a scarf. Ask first patient of each pair to move a scarf to the music while the second patient uses a scarf to imitate the movement. Follow by having the patients switch roles (i.e., the second patient assumes the first patient's role and the first patient assumes the second patient's role) so the imitation skills of all patients can be observed. M-41; F-41

Select one patient to lead the group in a creative movement activity. Observe whether each group member follows the leader's movements to music. M-32

NL-2 Changes movement in response to music ($n^3 = 1$; $n^4 = 1$; $n^5 = 2$; 22.22%)

Use a parachute activity in which short musical excerpts are used to accompany the movement of the parachute. Ask the patient to respond to different musical styles by moving the parachute in a manner that reflects the mood, rhythm and tempo of the music. M-41; F-41

NL-3 Taps fingers on legs or tray, taps toes, or claps to music ($n^3 = 1$; $n^4 = 1$; $n^5 = 2$; 22.22%)

Play patient-preferred music, or "patient-era" music if the patient's musical preferences are unknown. Lively instrumental music is recommended because music with lyrics may be distracting. M-40

Observe rhythmic response to music during group or one-to-one session (e.g., tapping fingers, toes, or clapping). F-36

NL-4 Follows and maintains pulse; claps in rhythm to the beat of the music ($n^3 = 1$; $n^4 = 1$; $n^5 = 2$; 22.22%)

Play recorded music, or the piano, and observe whether the resident can clap his hands to the beat of the music. M-25

The therapist models the rhythmic beat (e.g., finger snaps or claps) and the patient continues independently. Observe the patient's ability to follow the therapist and maintain the tempo. F-32

CHAPTER 7

ADOLESCENTS – MUSIC BEHAVIOR

(N = 104; 100%)

ASSESSMENT AREA – LISTENING TO MUSIC
(n = 30; 28.85%)

BEHAVIOR

L-1 Demonstrates awareness of a variety of styles of music rather than a single style (e.g., prefers only the latest teenage "sensation"); demonstrates musical knowledge; can discuss musical likes and dislikes using musical terms; tolerates the music preferences of others rather than becoming aggressive toward others because of their musical preferences; is not opinionated about musical preferences to the extent of being intolerant of the preferences of others; gains awareness of the discipline of composition; learns to respect both past and present composers (n^1 = 11; 36.67%)

MUSIC THERAPY INTERVENTION

At the beginning of the session, greet the patients with an opening song. 35

Conduct a "rate a record" session in which each group member rates their preference for each group member's chosen song. 50

Ask the patients to each choose a song that best describes themselves and to play the song for the group. Follow with a discussion of why the song describes the patient, and why the patient likes the song. 50

If the patient prefers only one type of music, conduct a lyric analysis. Ask the patient to describe the meaning of the lyrics and to tell why she likes the music. 45

Construct a music listening schedule to provide each patient the opportunity to listen to their preferred music. 45

Listen to a variety of music. After each composition is played, analyze the style of music, musical form, the rhythm, the chord structure, and whether the composition was a vocal or instrumental performance. Have each patient explain why they did or did not like the music. Note whether the preference expressed was because of the musical characteristics or because of another reason. 43-40-50

Play a variety of music for the adolescent music therapy group. After each selection is played ask a group member to give feedback relating to the music. Encourage each patient to give positive feedback, or to give at least one positive comment for every negative comment. 40

Study the lives and works of famous composers with the students. Listen to the compositions and assist the students in understanding what each composer is "trying to say" musically. 50

Without playing the music, give the patients the lyrics to a variety of unfamiliar music and ask them to pick out the lyrics of a song that is meaningful, or that relates to their life. After discussing the lyrics, have them listen to the music. Foster the realization that songs they don't normally listen to can be meaningful to them. 40

L-2   Demonstrates musical preferences ($n^1 = 9$; 30.00%)

During "free listening" let each patient choose their favorite song to play for the group then explain their choice. 50

Ask the patients to bring taped music that expresses their opinion about a topic chosen by the group. Observe each patient's music preferences as well as their tolerance for the music preferences of others. 31

Observe whether the patient makes "healthy" music choices, or "unhealthy" music choices that reinforce inappropriate behavior. Conduct lyric analysis to examine the patient's music preferences. 46

During music appreciation, conduct the "rate-a-record" activity in which each patient rates their musical preferences. Develop the patient's awareness of how listening to specific types of music can influence a person socially, mentally and physically. 46

Involve the patient in a "rate-a-record" session during which recordings are played, then rated and discussed by each patient. 40

Given an extensive list of songs, ask the patient to choose a song from the list to play for the group. Follow by asking the patient why she likes the song and what the song means to her. 40

Ask each patient to bring a song to play for the group at the next session. 35

Play a variety of music and ask the patients to state their opinion of the music. 50

THERAPIST NOTE: The adolescent's "rock music world" is highly significant in regard to affective and interpersonal issues. 50

L-3   Listens to or uses music for own physical and emotional relaxation; develops an awareness of various classical and jazz styles used for relaxation ($n^1 = 2$; 6.67%)

In the presence of relaxing background music, ask the patients to relax, to surround themselves by their favorite color, and to create a "safe place" in their imagination. 50

Conduct progressive muscle relaxation and guided imagery to jazz or classical background music. 40

L-4 Demonstrates the ability to associate affect with corresponding music; verbalizes perceived mood of preferred music; identifies the mood of the music ($n^1 = 1$; 3.33%)

Ask the group members to bring to the music therapy session four songs, each corresponding to a specific feeling, such as "happy," "sad," "mad," or "scared." Play the songs and have the group discuss which emotion category would be appropriate for each song. 36

L-5 Exhibits interest in new areas of music ($n^1 = 1$; 3.33%)

Conduct a discussion of current musical trends, new innovations in musical equipment, and the latest music technology. 31

L-6 Chooses music that expresses own social, political, interpersonal, and religious viewpoints ($n^1 = 1$; 3.33%)

Ask the patients to bring to the session taped music which expresses their opinion about a topic chosen by the group. 31

L-7 Demonstrates the ability to identify differences in timbre, pitch, and the overall mood of music ($n^1 = 1$; 3.33%)

Ask the patient to draw or write while focusing on a feeling in the presence of background music. 50

L-8 Develops confidence in the validity of own musical interpretations ($n^1 = 1$; 3.33%)

Have the students listen to an instrumental piece, then write and discuss their thoughts, images, and ideas of the meaning of the piece. 40

L-9 Listens to the lyrics of music ($n^1 = 1$; 3.33%)

During lyric discussion, study the lives of both past and present composers. Study the songs or works of composers who were successful despite overwhelming odds and great obstacles. 50

L-10 Concentrates on entire music composition while listening; attends to music ($n^1 = 1$; 3.33%)

Observe the patient's ability to concentrate on, attend to, or listen to music compositions during music listening. If the patient experiences apparent difficulty, ask the patient to listen to one particular musical element (e.g., a particular music instrument). It may be necessary to start with listening assignments of short duration, then to gradually lengthen the duration of the assignments as the patient masters them. 40

PLAYING INSTRUMENTS
(n = 19; 18.27%)

BEHAVIOR

P-1 Patient demonstrates an interest in music; expresses a desire to play an instrument (n^1 = 8; 42.12%)

MUSIC THERAPY INTERVENTION

Involve the patients in group activities where various aspects of music are demonstrated. For example, provide demonstrations of keyboards, the guitar, recording techniques, drums (trap set), string bass, electronic and computerized musical equipment, and MIDI. Conduct structured rhythmic and melodic activities using the instruments. Note whether the patient follows instructions in the proper use of instruments. 31-40-50

Involve the patient in a rhythmic activity using Kodály notation. 50

Provide patients with the opportunity to take lessons on instruments they are interested in. Encourage daily practice. 31-45

Establish goals that are motivating and challenging. Grade students weekly on progress toward these goals (e.g., David will play "Stairway to Heaven" on guitar; David will play the "C" major and "G" major scales three octaves). 50

Work individually with each student to assure success in meeting their musical goals. Also, provide a much needed "therapeutic ear." For example during individual lessons, David, a student, may speak about suicide. Discuss this openly with David and quickly get professional help for him. 50

P-2 Plays instrument for others; possesses music skill, talent, or training (n^1 = 6; 31.58%)

Invite the patient to perform for the therapist or the group. Observe the patient's ability to control possible performance anxiety. If performance anxiety is manifest, give the patient additional experience at performing before other group members during the music therapy session. The group performances should be the decision of the patient. If the patient has the skill to perform but does not desire to perform for others, then the music therapist should increase the patient's self confidence during individual music lessons. Performance material could include music learned from private lessons with the music therapist. Discuss with the patient any feelings of performance anxiety both before and after his or her recital. 31-50

Ask the patient to bring to the therapy session music that they have previously learned. Observe degree of musical training or talent. 50

Provide the patient with an opportunity to play an instrument in the talent show or other special events. 51

Involve the patient in an ensemble. Have the ensemble rehearse a patient-preferred song such as "Right Stuff" by New Kids on the Block. After learning the song, have the ensemble first perform for one or two staff, and then for the hospital dance. 46

Invite each student to audition for the "Student of the Month" assembly in which the school recognizes academic and behavioral achievement. The auditions require intensive preparation. Appoint a panel of two staff and two students to judge the auditions. If three of the four judges accept the audition as passing, the student gets to give the "Student of the Month" performance. 50

P-3 Participates in a group ensemble; cooperates and blends with the group; demonstrates musical sensitivity; is not excessively demanding (e.g., must always be the soloist) (n^1 = 2; 10.53%)

Have the ensemble perform a preferred composition, such as "Right Stuff" by New Kids on the Block. Let the patients take turns directing the ensemble. Note whether each patient is able to direct the tempo, dynamics and the soloists, to identify musical elements, and to give and receive suggestions for an improved performance. 40-46

P-4 Critiques musical performance; gives and receives constructive criticism or opinions (n^1 = 1; 5.26%)

Following a live or recorded performance of the group ensemble, prompt the patients to express their opinions about the performance. 40

P-5 Demonstrates rhythmic ability sufficient to play an instrument (n^1 = 1; 5.26%)

Involve the patient in a rhythmic imitation activity in which the therapist plays a short rhythm and the patient imitates. If the patient successfully imitates, do a follow-up activity in which the therapist plays a 12-bar blues pattern while the patient provides a rhythmic accompaniment. 35

P-6 Develops respect for various musical styles by participating in instrumental ensembles (n^1 = 1; 5.26%)

Have the group instrumental ensemble play a variety of music, such as African music, blues, gospel, spirituals, and jazz. 40

IMPROVISING MUSIC
(n = 17; 16.35%)

BEHAVIOR

I-1 Varies improvisation by changing the pitch, the rhythm, and the volume (n^1 = 4; 23.53%)

MUSIC THERAPY INTERVENTION

Observe the patient's ability to imitate changes in pitch, rhythm and volume while improvising. Play "Musical Duets" in which one patient leads the improvisation while the other patient imitates. 50

Give the patient a xylophone or metallophone and ask the patient to play any notes he or she wishes to play as the therapist accompanies with a rhythmic ostinato. Note the range of notes the patient plays. 46

Ask the patients to each choose an instrument. The therapist then begins an improvisation. Each group member, upon feeling comfortable enough, joins in the improvisation using their chosen instrument. Observe the quality of each patient's improvisation in terms of melody, pitch, rhythm, intensity, and creativity. 50

Given melodic Orff instruments with only the bars to the pentatonic scale, ask the patient to play three different instruments in three different ways (without being destructive) while the therapist plays an ostinato pattern on a bass instrument. The total performance should last approximately two minutes. Observe the patient's ability to perform contrasting improvisations. 46

I-2 Demonstrates the ability to improvise on a melodic instrument within a rhythmic structure; able to improvise rhythmic patterns (n^1 = 3; 17.65%)

Have the patient improvise on a metallophone while the group provides an ostinato rhythmic accompaniment on percussion instruments. This condition also may be implemented utilizing a variety of percussion instruments. 40-43

During improvisation, observe the patient's ability to improvise on progressively more complex harmonic structures (e.g., pentatonic, blues, rock 'n roll, or popular). 40

I-3 Demonstrates awareness of the musical responses of other group members during improvisational activities; listens to the improvisations of other group members to produce a blending and cohesive sound during group improvisation (n^1 = 2; 11.77%)

During group improvisation ask one patient to conduct or lead the group improvisation. Observe the improvisations of each group member. 50

During structured improvisation, ask the patients to do a group improvisation of a word or a feeling. 50

I-4 Demonstrates an interest in playing music instruments; realizes instant success ($n^1 = 2$; 11.77%)

Arrange for the patient to improvise on a variety of instruments. 50

Ask the students to improvise various feelings or situations on their preferred instruments. Encourage interest and motivation by letting the students discover they can experiment and improvise on instruments without having to take lessons. 40

I-5 Demonstrates the ability to improvise on the pentatonic scale ($n^1 = 2$; 11.77%)

Provide the patient with the notes of the pentatonic scale using the xylophone or tone bells. Prompt the patient to improvise on the pentatonic scale (e.g., "Play some different five-note patterns."). 35-50

I-6 Improvises on the blues scale; discovers a means of self expression by playing, singing, and improvising in blues style ($n^1 = 1$; 5.88%)

Teach the patients the basic structure of the blues, then have them improvise both instrumentally and vocally in blues form and style. 40

I-7 Demonstrates the ability to create improvisations representative of moods ($n^1 = 1$; 5.88%)

Ask the patient to improvise a current feeling. 50

I-8 Demonstrates the ability to improvise with one other person ($n^1 = 1$; 5.88%)

Select two patients and give each a xylophone with only the tone bars forming the pentatonic scale. Ask the patients to work together at improvising a musical composition. 43

I-9 Improvises musically rather than randomly playing notes on an instrument ($n^1 = 1$; 5.88%)

Introduce to the patient simple rhythmic and melodic patterns. Suggest and demonstrate simple improvisatory techniques. 45

I-10 Improvises movement to music (see "Participates in unstructured creative movement to music" under "Locomotor Movement to Music")

SINGING
(n = 17; 16.35%)

BEHAVIOR

| S-1 | Observe singing skills such as the ability to match pitch and follow rhythms (n^1 = 4; 23.53%) |

MUSIC THERAPY INTERVENTION

Conduct a sing-a-long. Observe the patient singing. 50

Play middle "C" on the piano and ask the patient to sing the pitch. 46

Note each patient's most comfortable pitch. Ask each patient to sing their most comfortable pitch, then match the pitch using the piano. 46

Observe the patient's ability to sing a melody with rhythmic and melodic accuracy. Ask the patient to sing a familiar popular song while the therapist plays the melody. 46

| S-2 | Sings solo in front of group (n^1 = 3; 17.65%) |

Conduct the Alphabet Game. Ask the patients to name a song for each letter of the alphabet. Give bonus points to patients for singing a song phrase or a song before the group. 50

Provide the patient with an opportunity to sing in the talent show or other special events. 40-51

| S-3 | Blends with group when singing; does not sing louder than other group members (n^1 = 3; 17.65%) |

Videotape the "Music Show" rehearsal during each music therapy session. When viewing the videotape, assist patients in understanding the importance of blending with the other group members and in presenting a group effort. 36

During choir rehearsal, encourage the patients to listen to their own singing, to each other, and to follow or match the conductor's cues. 31

Observe the patient singing a solo or singing with the group. 40

| S-4 | Sings with adequate loudness; does not sing with a low inaudible voice (n^1 = 2; 11.77%) |

Involve the patient, who does not sing loudly enough, in a chorus or in group singing. The patient may sing as loud as the other group members, which may in turn strengthen the patient's voice. 40-36

S-5 Sings with a vocal tone that is not too breathy (n^1 = 1; 5.88%)

If the patient's vocal tone is too breathy when singing, tape record the patient's singing each session to stimulate her awareness of how she sounds. 36

S-6 Sings in tune with a pleasing timbre (n^1 = 1; 5.88%)

Observe the patient singing a solo or singing with the group. 40

S-7 Sings with proper diction (n^1 = 1; 5.88%)

Involve the patient in group singing in which the group members are called upon to sing impromptu solos. 36

S-8 Demonstrates expanded vocal range resulting in increased confidence in singing ability (n^1 = 1; 5.88%)

Conduct vocal warm-ups at the beginning of each choir rehearsal to establish or expand singing range. 31

S-9 Sings with a choir (n^1 = 1; 5.88%)

Give patients the opportunity to sing in a choir. Schedule the choir to perform every two or three months. Discuss with the choir feelings about performance anxiety both before and after each choir concert. 31

COMPOSING MUSIC
(n = 17; 16.35%)

BEHAVIOR

C-1 Demonstrates the ability to write music including lyrics and melody; composes and performs own music; demonstrates the ability to compose lyrics and phrases that fit the rhythm of the song; is able to use music composition as a means of self expression (n^1 = 4; 23.53%)

MUSIC THERAPY INTERVENTION

Assist the patients in writing lyrics that are based on a topic chosen by the music therapist. Following a discussion of musical style, have the group choose a style, then write a melody in the chosen style that matches the lyrics. Emotionally disturbed students often have "more to say" emotionally than do "normal" students. 40-43-50

During group song writing, write a song, lyrics, and rhythmic accompaniment which is based on current treatment or unit issues. 50

C-2   Develops the ability to use lyric writing as a means of self expression; writes own lyrics (n^1 = 3; 17.65%)

Introduce various lyric or song writing techniques, such as fill-in-the-blank, blues form, parody, and song writing. THERAPIST NOTE: One of our students wrote lyrics meaningful enough to be reviewed by the American Psychiatric Association (APA). 40-40-50

C-3   Participates in writing song parodies (n^1 = 2; 11.76%)

After identifying a patient-preferred song, individualize the song by having the patient either rewrite all the lyrics or rewrite only part of the lyrics (e.g., rewrite a key word for each phrase: "Fill in the blank."). Using the melody of a familiar song, have the patient write new lyrics which describe herself and her experiences. 43-46

C-4   Participates in music composition activities in which compositions are based on pictures, themes, or abstract objects or symbols (e.g., lightning, water, the Sun, an exclamation mark [!], unfamiliar instrumental music) (n^1 = 2; 11.76%)

Have the patients listen to a recording used for guided imagery. After listening to the composition, have the patients elaborate on and develop the guided imagery composition using Orff instruments, chants, movement, and music composition techniques. 40

Given a theme such as "Stay in School," have the group compose a composition or rap based on the theme. Select the theme within specified guidelines, create the rhymes or raps, add percussion, perform, and record. 40

C-5   Experiences difficulty with composing song lyrics because of the inability to respond rhythmically (n^1 = 2; 11.76%)

Assist the patient with composing and establishing a rhythm. Once the rhythm is learned, assist the patient in creating a rap song based on the rhythm (e.g., My name is _____. I'm here to say _____ today. [to an accompanying rhythm]). 36-46

C-6   Demonstrates respect for a variety of musical styles (n^1 = 1; 5.88%)

Have the students write a song (lyrics and music) combining two styles of music. 40

C-7   Has trouble rhyming or thinking of lyrics for phrases because of a poor vocabulary (n^1 = 1; 5.88%)

Play a song that can be used as a parody. Give the patient a copy of the song lyrics and assist the patient in deleting certain parts of speech, such as the nouns, adjectives, or clauses. The patient then substitutes new words for the deleted words, changing the meaning of the song. 36

C-8 Demonstrates the ability to use imagination to create music productions (n^1 = 1; 5.88%)

Involve the patients in creating their own music video and radio productions. 40

C-9 Demonstrates the ability to organize sounds into music (n^1 = 1; 5.88%)

Let each group member choose an instrument to play, and let one patient serve as the conductor. The conductor's responsibility is to direct the rhythm, the melody, the instrumentation and other musical characteristics to compose a musical composition. 43

LOCOMOTOR MOVEMENT TO MUSIC
(n = 4; 3.85%)

BEHAVIOR

LM-1 Participates in unstructured creative movement to music; improvises movement to music; moves creatively to music (n^1 = 2; 50.00%)

MUSIC THERAPY INTERVENTION

Assess the patient's spontaneous movement to music. Use patient-preferred music. 35

In the presence of music, assist the patients in creating a movement pattern, and then in memorizing the movement pattern. If working with a large group of patients, split the group into two or three smaller groups and have each patient take a turn performing the movement (e.g., round robin format). 43

LM-2 Dances the latest dance styles to preferred music (e.g., rap music; the latest teenage "sensation") (n^1 = 1; 25.00%)

Use the above dances to promote therapeutic goals (e.g., exercise, group leadership through demonstrating or teaching others to dance, self-expressiveness, group cohesiveness, and peer acceptance). 45

LM-3 Has trouble dancing because of the inability to respond to cues (n^1 = 1; 25.00%)

Assist the patient in establishing a dance routine with which she can be successful (e.g., four to six individual movements). Have the patient repeat the routine to the count of eight. 36

CHAPTER 8

CHILDREN – MUSIC BEHAVIOR

(N = 57; 100%)

ASSESSMENT AREA – LISTENING TO MUSIC
(n = 14; 24.56%)

BEHAVIOR

L-1 Demonstrates the ability to identify characteristics of music, such as musical style, which instruments are playing, the tempo of the music (i.e., slow or fast), and whether the selection is an instrumental or vocal; recognizes a variety of musical styles; listens discriminatively to music (n^1 = 8; 57.14%)

MUSIC THERAPY INTERVENTION

During music listening, have the patient identify the name of the musical selection, the style of music, the instrumentation, whether the tempo is slow or fast, whether the dynamics are loud or soft, whether the selection is an instrumental or vocal. If the selection was a vocal ask the patient whether a man or woman was singing. Adjust the task to the capability of the patient. 20-20-36-40

After listening to each musical selection, ask the patient to state whether or not they liked the musical style and why. 36

Play Instrument Bingo. This game is played the same as the usual game of Bingo with the exception that the "calls" are short excerpts of certain instruments playing. The child is asked to place a chip on the corresponding picture of the instrument that is playing (Note: Sounds of instruments may be obtained from the recording, "A Young Person's Guide to the Orchestra," Opus 32 [Britten, 1946]. Also recordings of common instruments such as piano, guitar, autoharp, and percussion instruments may be used). 40

Teach the patient to identify the names of music instruments. Present to the patient flash cards, each with a picture of a music instrument and the name of the music instrument. Teach the patient to pronounce and spell by rote the name of the music instrument. Monitor the patient's correct responses. 50

Teach the patient to identify instruments by family grouping, emphasizing the distinguishing characteristics of each family of instruments. 50

L-2 Demonstrates the ability to choose preferred music, or to state musical preferences (n^1 = 2; 14.29%)

Play a variety of music and ask the patient to rate the songs in order of preference. Provide assistance when needed. 40

The patient will choose a song for music listening from a variety of record albums. 20

L-3   Reads the lyrics to songs (n^1 = 2; 14.29%)

Give the patients a copy of the lyrics to a song. Observe the ability of the patients to read the lyrics; provide assistance if needed. 50

Give the patients a copy of the lyrics to a song. Observe the ability of the patients to follow the lyrics as the song is playing. After the song ends, conduct a discussion of the content of the lyrics and of the patients' interpretation of the lyrics. 50

L-4   Identifies popular songs (n^1 = 1; 7.14%)

Play the game, Name That Tune. 40

L-5   Demonstrates audience behavior appropriate to a variety of live music (n^1 = 1; 7.14%)

Take patients on periodic field trips to attend live informal music performances (i.e., jazz, pop concert, street music, dance music). 20

SINGING
(n = 14; 24.56%)

BEHAVIOR

S-1   Sings on pitch; matches pitch; sings in tune (n^1 = 4; 28.57%)

MUSIC THERAPY INTERVENTION

Observe the patient singing various children's songs. 86

Before singing a song, the therapist sings the first pitch of the song and the patient matches the pitch. 40

Observe the patient singing a cappella, a song of choice. 40

Ask the patient to sing a familiar song. The therapist chooses the song to be sung and provides an instrumental accompaniment using the piano or guitar. 40

S-2   Sings melodic phrases; sings lyrics to songs (n^1 = 4; 28.57%)

Sing several melodic phrases for the patient. After each phrase, ask the patient to sing an imitation or duplication of the phrase. 51

Teach the patient a song one line at a time by rote (the therapist sings a line, then the patient imitates). 36

Ask the patient to spontaneously sing a solo as a special feature during group singing. 56

The therapist models phrase by phrase the correct articulation of the song lyrics. After each phrase, the patients repeat the lyrics back to the therapist. This exercise is done without singing, with the rhythmic character of a chant. Body rhythms or rhythm instruments may be utilized to accompany the recitations. Following this exercise, teach the patients to sing the lyrics with the correct inflection, pitch, and intonation. Use the same technique as above with the exception that the patients sing each phrase after it is modeled by the therapist. 50

S-3   Sings with music therapist from a song book ($n^1 = 2$; 14.29%)

Have the patient choose from a song book a familiar song to sing. The therapist and the patient will then sing the song together. Note the patient's ability to begin and end the song on time, and the ability to maintain the tempo. 33

When discussing familiar songs, observe the child's emotional response. Does the child exhibit facial expressions such as sadness or joy? 33

S-4   Sings from the beginning to the end of a song without being distracted ($n^1 = 1$; 7.14%)

Ask the patient to perform in the center of the group as the "guest singer." Observe the patient's ability to sing without becoming distracted. 56

S-5   Sings loudly enough to be heard by an audience ($n^1 = 1$; 7.14%)

Prepare the patients to sing in a music show. During rehearsals, tape record the patients singing the music for the music show, then have them sing along with the tape recording. Challenge the patients to sing as loud as the tape recording. 56

S-6   Chooses songs from song book that are reminiscent of family members ($n^1 = 1$; 7.14%)

During group discussion ask the children to select a song that reminds them of their family members. Read with the children the song titles in the table of contents. Observe each child's response to the song title topics. Does the child avoid or retreat from songs that remind her of various family members? 33

S-7   Sings a song from memory ($n^1 = 1$; 7.14%)

Ask the patient to sing a familiar song from memory. The therapist may sing along with the patient. Observe the content and mood of the song the patient chooses. 33

PLAYING INSTRUMENTS
(n = 11; 19.30%)

BEHAVIOR

P-1 Responds rhythmically to music; responds to music by keeping a rhythmic pulse (n^1 = 2; 18.18%)

MUSIC THERAPY INTERVENTION

During rhythm band group, have each patient play a rhythm that coincides with a rhythm performed by another patient. 56

During music listening, ask the patient to clap her hands, nod her head, and/ or tap her foot in response to a variety of musical selections and tempi. 20

P-2 Plays a variety of instruments (n^1 = 2; 18.18%)

Give the patient the opportunity to play a variety of instruments, such as bar (Orff) instruments, guitar or autoharp, recorder, electronic keyboard, and the drum machine. 40

Have each child play a variety of Orff instruments in a pentatonic ensemble. 36

P-3 Plays instrument on cue; follows musical cues (n^1 = 1; 9.09%)

Ask the patient to play a rhythm instrument to a song at pre-specified times as indicated by the therapist's cue. Observe the patient's ability to start and stop playing on cue. 40

P-4 Plays autoharp; uses a class room instrument to accompany a musical selection (n^1 = 1; 9.09%)

Invite the patient to participate with the music therapist in playing the auto-harp (e.g., the therapist presses the chords and sings as the patient strums the strings). Continue to teach basic skills necessary for playing the autoharp in-dependently. Observe the patient's memory ability, attention span, the ability to follow directions, and rhythmic ability. 33

P-5 Plays choir chimes (n^1 = 1; 9.09%)

Instruct the patient in the correct usage of choir chimes (e.g., holding and ringing the choir chimes). To reinforce correct usage, have the patients play from charts (choir chime music) of preferred songs. NOTE: For an example of choir chime or hand bell music, see Rubin (1976). 50

P-6 Plays guitar (n^1 = 1; 9.09%)

Using nontraditional Multichord guitar technique (Cassity, 1977), play a blues progression in which each patient strums their guitar upon cue. 36

P-7   Uses rhythm/lumi sticks correctly ($n^1 = 1$; 9.09%)

Instruct the patient in the correct usage of rhythm/lumi sticks. Use call and response activities to give the patient experience in the correct usage of the sticks. 50

P-8   Listens to tape recording of own instrumental performance ($n^1 = 1$; 9.09%)

Tape record the group's instrumental performance, then have the group listen to the tape following the performance. 36

P-9   Plays music instrument for peer or staff member ($n^1 = 1$; 9.09%)

Ask the child to choose a favorite staff person with whom to share her newly acquired autoharp performance skills. Assess the child's relationship with authority figures in terms of which staff is chosen, and how she responds to the staff person. 33

LOCOMOTOR MOVEMENT TO MUSIC
($n = 8$; 14.04%)

BEHAVIOR

LM-1   Creates movements to music; performs unstructured creative movement ($n^1 = 2$; 25.00%)

MUSIC THERAPY INTERVENTION

Play music that has a danceable rhythm or a clearly defined beat. Ask the patient to create a movement to the music. Observe the degree of expressiveness exhibited while moving to the music. 36-40

LM-2   Participates in choreography ($n^1 = 1$; 12.50%)

Teach the patient the steps to a choreographed movement. Note the ability of the patient to remember the dance sequence. Proceed from easy to more difficult choreography. 40

LM-3   Imitates or mirrors musical movement ($n^1 = 1$; 12.50%)

Play music of a danceable quality. Ask the patient to imitate the musical movement of the therapist or a peer. 36

LM-4   Moves in rhythm to the music; follows directions for movement ($n^1 = 1$; 12.50%)

Observe the ability of the children to perform body action songs. For example, play the song, "Sally the Swinging Snake" and encourage the children to move to the music and to do the actions described in the song. 40

LM-5 Moves freely and spontaneously without rigidity (n^1 = 1; 12.50%)

If the patient exhibits rigidity in movement, start by involving the patient in marching exercises. Prepare the patient to eventually participate in creative movement depicting environment objects such as animals. 56

LM-6 Follows sequence of movement activity (n^1 = 1; 12.50%)

If the patient has difficulty following the sequence of a movement activity, involve the patient in number games in which each child must respond when her number is sung (e.g., Have the patients relate numbers to objects while singing songs such as "Ten Little Pennies (Indians)," "This Old Man," and "Three Little Speckled Frogs." [Cassity, 1985]). 56

LM-7 Walks to the beat of the music (n^1 = 1; 12.50%)

Ask the patients to walk in a circle to the beat of a drum. Vary the tempo of the beat and observe whether the patients alter their walking pace to match the tempo of the drum beat. 36

COMPOSING MUSIC
(n = 4; 7.02%)

BEHAVIOR

C-1 Composes new lyrics to songs; composes a parody; participates in lyric substitution activities (n^1 = 3; 75.00%)

MUSIC THERAPY INTERVENTION

Give the patient experience at composing lyrics to fit the established melodic and rhythmic limits of a song. 33

Using a song which has a topic the child considers to be nonthreatening, observe the child's ability to suggest lyrics that fit rhythmically into the song phrases. Also note the complexity of words the child chooses and the accuracy of their meaning. 33

Using a song which has a topic relating to the child's problems, observe the child's ability to suggest lyrics that fit rhythmically into the song phrases. Note the child's level of insight into her problems and her assessment of the situation. 33

C-2 Composes a greeting song (n^1 = 1; 25.00%)

Have each patient decide how many beats her name is. For example, Mar-ga-ret would be three beats. Next ask each patient to choose an Orff instrument on which to play each beat of her name. Give each patient the choice of three instruments. Next write each patient's name, the chosen instrument, and the rhythmic and melodic notation of her name on an adapted music staff. Finally have the group sing a standard greeting song, with each group member playing her name at the appropriate time (e.g., Hel-lo Margaret, Hel-lo Margaret, Hel-lo Margaret, we're glad you're here today [to the tune of "Good Night Ladies"]). 36

IMPROVISING MUSIC
(n = 2; 3.51%)

BEHAVIOR

I-1   Uses improvisation to create a song (n^1 = 1; 50.00%)

MUSIC THERAPY INTERVENTION

Give the patient experience at setting limits necessary to create a song. Assist the patient in creating a song by improvising with instruments, body percussion, or their voice. 36

I-2   Directs the performance of an improvised song (n^1 = 1; 50.00%)

After creating a song have the patient conduct the song, directing when each instrument will play and what instrument will play. 36

NONLOCOMOTOR MOVEMENT TO MUSIC
(n = 4; 7.02%)

BEHAVIOR

NL-1   Claps rhythms; remembers and reproduces rhythms accurately (n^1 = 4; 100%)

MUSIC THERAPY INTERVENTION

Ask the patients to take turns mirroring each other's rhythmic clapping. 86

Clap several rhythms for the patient. After each rhythm is clapped, ask the patient to clap an imitation or duplication of the rhythm. 51

Play the game, Telephone. This game is played by first dividing the children into pairs so that each child has a partner. Each child will "transmit a message" to her partner by tapping the rhythmic sequence of the message on her partner's back. The partner will acknowledge the message by repeating the tapped rhythm on the child's back. The partner is then given one minute to guess what the message was. The child may assist her partner by only using gestures or nonverbal communication. Words are not allowed. If the partner cannot guess the message within one minute the child and the partner lose a point. The partners with the most points win. 40

Part III

PRACTICE EXERCISES
GROUP THERAPY
BRIEF THERAPY

CHAPTER 9

PRACTICE EXERCISES

Multimodal music therapy corresponds closely to the *Standards of Clinical Practice* of the American Music Therapy Association (AMTA, 1998) in terms of accountability. Following is an illustration of how each element of the AMTA *General Standards* corresponds to the multimodal music therapy accountability procedure.

AMTA General Standards	Multimodal Music Therapy Procedure
1. Referral and Acceptance	1. Provides specific initial information about the patient to facilitate the decision of whether to accept.
2. Assessment	2. Administer PMTQ; review results of other assessments; consult with other professionals; construct a BASIC I.D.
3. Program Planning	3. Construct the Multimodal Music Therapy Profile and a Music Therapy Intervention Plan for each goal.
4. Implementation	4. Write an Implementation Strategy for achieving each objective.
5. Documentation	5. Maintain a Music Therapy Progress Report Chart for each objective.
6. Termination of Services	6. Provides objective evidence of whether therapy should be terminated. If so, provides adequate documentation for preparation of termination plan.

For the assessment phase the Standards mandate the assessment of the patient's (1) non-music behavior or problems, (2) music behavior, and (3) strengths and needs. The PMTQ assesses all three, with strengths and needs indicated by the PMTQ rating scale. The PMTQ also is appropriate for the patient's chronological age (a separate PMTQ is provided for each chronological age level), and level of functioning (GAF ratings are requested in the PMTQ; the music therapy interventions in this manual have GAF ratings) as required by the Standards.

For the program planning phase the Standards require that the program plan be individualized, indicate the type, frequency, and duration of music therapy involvement, specify goals and operationally defined objectives, specify procedures, and provide for periodic evaluation and periodic modification. All these requirements are met by multimodal music therapy. The clinical forms in Appendix IV provide for the recording of all the above information.

Of all the above stages of accountability, assessment is most crucial. In the absence of an adequate assessment one cannot successfully meet the patient's needs in terms of program planning, implementation, or documentation. Conducting an adequate assessment therefore is the *sine qua non* of every music therapy program. A major component of the assessment phase in multimodal music therapy is the PMTQ. The ability to accurately administer and interpret the PMTQ is very important if multimodal music therapy is to be successfully implemented. The following exercises therefore are designed to give the reader experience at analyzing the PMTQ to determine patient problems for purposes of program planning. The reader should study Chapter 2 thoroughly before attempting to do the following exercises.

Instructions for PMTQ Analysis

The purpose of the following exercises is to provide experience at analyzing information in a completed PMTQ. Following are four PMTQs containing information about psychiatric patients. From information in each PMTQ, do the following:

1. Construct a *BASIC I.D.*
2. Construct a *Multimodal Music Therapy Profile* from information in the above BASIC-I.D.
3. Write one *Music Therapy Intervention Plan* for each goal.
4. Write one *Implementation Strategy* for each objective that you wrote in Step 3.
5. Use a *Music Therapy Progress Report Chart* to chart hypothetical progress. You will need to write one Music Therapy Progress Report Chart for each objective you wrote in Step 3.

It is very important to note whether your PMTQ is designed for adults, adolescents, or children so you can refer to the appropriate section of the manual to obtain the problems and interventions appropriate for the chronological age level of your patient. You also will need to use the Multimodal Music Therapy Profile form that is appropriate for the age level of your patient (Appendix IV).

Extra clinical forms for writing the above music therapy treatment plans may be found in Appendix IV. You will need to copy these forms so you can keep the originals for future use. Be sure to check your work with the case examples of *D, M, B,* and *J* given in Chapter 2. Note especially the correct format for writing goals and objectives, and how the same goals and objectives are evaluated in the progress report chart.

If you are in a classroom situation the following procedure could be used:

1. Divide the class into four groups. Assign each group to write a treatment plan based on one of the following completed *PMTQs*.

2. The members of each group work together to analyze their assigned PMTQ to produce a *BASIC I.D.* and a *Multimodal Music Therapy Profile*.

3. Each group member individually writes a *Music Therapy Intervention Plan* containing a goal and objectives based on the PMTQ analysis conducted in Step 2. The result is one Music Therapy Intervention Plan written by each member of the group with each Intervention Plan containing a different goal.

4. Each group member individually writes one *Implementation Strategy* for each objective he or she wrote in Step 3. For example, if the group member wrote three objectives, then she should write three implementation strategies.

5. Each group member completes one *Music Therapy Progress Report Chart* for each objective he or she wrote in Step 3. For example, if he or she wrote three objectives then there needs to be three Progress Report Charts. Be sure to write a hypothetical progress report for *each* session under *Session Progress Report/Comments* at the bottom of the Progress Report Chart.

6. If time permits, each group could report their final music therapy treatment plan to the class to simulate a music therapy report at a patient staffing. The presentation could include the results of the PMTQ analysis along with each group member's goals and objectives.

The reader may wish to use the following checklist to double check their work for completeness and accuracy:

	Task	Yes	No
1	Considers PMTQ items rated a *4* or *5* as problems.		
2	Aware that some PMTQ items are scored by reversing the scale.		
3	Uses letter-number references in PMTQ (e.g., A-5) to refer to detailed description of problems in this manual.		
4	Realizes that one or more PMTQ items can pertain to one letter-number.		
5	Aware of patient's chronological age level.		
6	Locates section in manual containing problems and interventions appropriate for the patient's chronological age.		
7	Transfers problems identified in PMTQ to BASIC I.D.		
8	Examines Post Interview Observations for additional problems.		
9	Uses Multimodal Music Therapy Profile appropriate for patient's chronological age.		
10	Writes name of client on the Multimodal Music Therapy Profile.		
11	Writes a narrative for the Multimodal Music Therapy Profile describing the patient's music preferences.		
12	Records letter-number of problems on the Multimodal Music Therapy Profile (e.g., A-2).		
13	Refers to BASIC I.D. to record problems on Multimodal Music Therapy Profile.		
14	Refers to appropriate section in manual or to patient preferences to write music therapy interventions.		
15	Writes a narrative in the Multimodal Music Therapy Profile describing the results of the PMTQ Post Interview Observations.		
16	Writes name of client on Music Therapy Intervention Plan (MTIP).		
17	Writes case number on MTIP.		
18	Writes date of assessment on MTIP (the date the PMTQ was administered).		
19	Writes the correct goal number (#) and goal name on the MTIP.		
20	Writes the goal statement on the MTIP.		
21	Writes the correct objective number (e.g., 1.2) on the MTIP.		
22	Writes operationally defined behavioral objectives consisting of conditions, observable behavior, and a measurable criterion. The target behaviors are focused on remediating problems in the BASIC I.D.		
23	Signs own name in MTIP after "Person Responsible."		
24	If objectives are actually implemented, records date started, date ended, and reason ended in MTIP.		

25	For Implementation Strategy (IS), writes name of patient, case number, and date of assessment.		
26	Writes objective number and specifies required materials in IS.		
27	Specifies reinforcement schedule (e.g., continuous, fixed, variable).		
28	Specifies kind of reinforcement (e.g., music, verbal, or both).		
29	Specifies detailed procedure in terms of therapist and patient behavior in IS.		
30	Writes agency's, patient's, and therapist's name in the Music Therapy Progress Report Chart (MTPRC).		
31	Specifies goal number and goal statement in the MTPRC.		
32	Specifies objective number and objective statement in MTPRC.		
33	Records date of each session in MTPRC.		
34	Records appropriate evaluation symbol to indicate progress.		
35	Writes a narrative progress report for each session.		

Common errors students make in achieving the above tasks are including two target behaviors in one objective, writing nonobservable target behaviors, writing goals and objectives that are musically oriented rather than therapeutically oriented (when the task is to target problems in the BASIC I.D.), writing criteria that are vague or unmeasurable, and an over reliance on one type of music therapy activity (e.g., lyric analysis) for no apparent reason. If, after checking your music therapy treatment plans with the above check list, you have questions about how to achieve the above tasks, review the examples provided in Chapter 2.

Adults: The case of Bob. The following PMTQ was administered to Bob, a lesbian female receiving music therapy services at the Southwestern Oklahoma State University Music Therapy Clinic. Bob was content with her homosexual life-style, and especially with her lesbian mate who served as a stable live-in and lover. However, Bob had other problems severe enough to warrant support services from the local mental health center. From information in Bob's PMTQ, construct a BASIC I.D., a multimodal music therapy profile, intervention plan(s), implementation strategy(ies), and chart hypothetical progress.

PATIENT IDENTIFICATION FORM

NAME: Bob _____   SEX: Female   AGE: 35 _____

FORMAL/PRIMARY DIAGNOSIS:

AXIS I: Schizophrenia, Paranoid Type (continuous) _____

AXIS II: Avoidant Personality Disorder _____

AXIS III: Seizure Disorder _____

AXIS IV: Estranged from family; unemployment. _____

AXIS V: Current GAF: 35 _____   Highest GAF past year: 40 _____

TOTAL NUMBER AND LENGTH OF STAYS OF PRIOR HOSPITALIZATIONS:

HOSPITAL	LENGTH OF STAY
Approximately 15 residential treatments	Unknown
statewide.	

LENGTH OF HOSPITALIZATION AT PRESENT FACILITY: NA (presently in community placement and outpatient treatment).

TYPES OF MEDICATION TAKEN	*AND* DOSAGE PRESCRIBED
Cogentin	2 mg twice daily
Haldol	5 mg 4 times daily

PSYCHIATRIC MUSIC THERAPY QUESTIONNAIRE
ADULTS

INSTRUCTIONS: Parts I and II of the following questionnaire are to be administered by the **examiner, or therapist, interviewing the examinee, or patient.** Part III, Post Interview Observations, will be completed by the examiner following termination of the interview, or Part II.

EXAMINER: A major purpose of therapy is to assist you with problems that may be interfering with your ability to enjoy life to the fullest. The purpose of this questionnaire therefore, is to assist you in recognizing problems or "bad habits" you may have and wish to get rid of. Since these questions are personal, you may be assured of complete confidentiality. NO ONE WILL SEE YOUR ANSWERS OTHER THAN THE THERAPISTS. If you do not care to answer these questions simply tell me you do not care to answer these questions.

I. MUSIC (viii)

1. EXAMINER: For the following styles of music tell me the number that indicates the degree you like each type of music. (Examiner gives the attached scale, like the one below, to the examinee.)

	Strongly Dislike	Dislike	Neutral	Like	Strongly Like
COUNTRY	1	2	③	4	5
POPULAR	1	2	3	④	5
ROCK	1	2	3	4	⑤
JAZZ	1	2	3	4	⑤
FOLK	1	2	③	4	5
RELIGIOUS	1	2	③	4	5
OTHER: *Classical*	1	2	3	4	⑤

2. EXAMINER: Who is your favorite performer or composer?
(INSTRUCTION: Examiner writes in name below)
Rock: Janice Joplin and Jimmy Hendrix; Classical: W. A. Mozart

INSTRUCTIONS FOR EXAMINER: Give the examinee the scale, like the one below, attached to this questionnaire. The examinee may then refer to the scale as necessary when choosing a number.

EXAMINER: I am going to read some statements. After each statement tell me the number from this scale that describes the extent you agree with the statement.

Strongly Disagree	Disagree	Neutral	Agree	Strongly Agree
1	2	3	4	5

3. _4_ I would like to participate in a group sing-a-long with a pianist or guitarist accompanying the group. (viii)

4. _2_ I would like to sing on stage before an audience.

5. _4_ I would like to learn to play a musical instrument.

II. MULTIMODAL PROBLEM ANALYSIS

INSTRUCTIONS FOR EXAMINER: Let the examinee continue to keep the scale, like the one below. The examinee may then refer to the scale as necessary when choosing a number.

EXAMINER: I am going to read some statements. After each statement tell me the number from this scale that describes the extent you agree with the statement.

Strongly Disagree	Disagree	Neutral	Agree	Strongly Agree
1	2	3	4	5

Interpersonal (iv)

1. _5_ I would rather be alone than be with people. (IS-1)

2. _3_ I find it hard to make friends.

3. _2_ I have no close friends.

4. _3_ It is easy for me to talk to people.

5. _4_ It is hard for me to talk when in a group of people.

6. _2_ I have trouble listening to others when they talk to me.

7. _2_ I do not have a hobby; I rarely do something just for fun. (IS-2, IS-4)

8. _3_ I would rather be alone or do nothing than to do something for fun with other people.

9. _2_ There is not much to do in my spare time other than to sleep or watch television.

10. _2_ I often get into trouble for not following directions, rules or regulations, or for not doing what I am suppose to do (e.g., smoking, eating, or drinking where prohibited). (IS-3)

11. _2_ Friendships or relationships with other people usually do not last more than one year. (IS-5)

12. _2_ I fight a lot with either my spouse (husband or wife) or family.

13. _3_ I would feel very uneasy telling a group of people my likes, dislikes, and personal experiences. (IS-6)

14. _4_ I have no difficulty being accepted by community groups (e.g., church, service groups) and with being invited to their events (e.g., parties, "get togethers"). (IS-7)

15. _2_ I would rather sit behind the group members or sit alone than to sit with the group. (IS-8)

16. _1_ I say the right things when trying to make friends with the opposite sex. (IS-9)

17. _2_ Listening to the problems of others is boring; I become impatient. (IS-10)

Affect (iii)

18. _5_ People cannot tell when I am happy, sad, or excited. (A-1)

19. _5_ I rarely feel happy, sad, excited, or smile.

20. _3_ I can easily tell when other people are happy, sad, or excited.

21. _3_ I never worry about anything. (A-2)

22. _1_ I never get angry or mad at people.

23. _5_ I frequently experience feelings of anger and stress (A-3)

24. _4_ I often hurt the feelings of my friends.

25. _5_ I often hit other people. (A-3, A-10)

26. _2_ I often feel like I have a tremendous amount of energy (i.e., difficulty sleeping, constantly moving and talking). (A-4)

27. _1_ I often feel like I have no energy and feel very sad. (A-5)

28. _2_ I frequently feel depressed or "down in the dumps."

29. _1_ I frequently feel like killing or hurting myself. (A-6)

30. _1_ I often wish I were dead.

31. _2_ I experience a lot of anxiety (A-7).

32. _3_ I often experience excessive anxiety from one or more of the following: present or past problems with other people, worry about the future (e.g., upcoming events), my life situation.

33. _2_ I often experience excessive anxiety that frequently results in one or more of the following: inability to relax, muscle stiffness, sleep disturbance, worry, verbally talking about my problems to myself or others.

34. _3_ It is easy for me to lose self-control and exhibit too much laughing, crying, or anger. (A-8)

35. _2_ I often become very, very scared along with one or more of the following: I get panicky, my heart beats fast, I experience shortness of breath. (A-9)

36. _2_ Sometimes I get so mad I could kill people. (A-10)

37. _5_ Sometimes I get so mad I hit people.

38. _5_ I frequently get mad when others give me advice.

39. _5_ People often tell me I have a bad temper.

Cognitive (iv)

40. _1_   I do not like myself. (C-1)
41. _2_   I frequently call myself names such as "stupid," "idiot," or "dumb."
42. _2_   I usually fail when I try to do something.
43. _3_   People like me.
44. _5_   I do not trust people. (C-2)
45. _4_   Other people frequently lie about me.
46. _2_   My problems are overwhelming; they can't be solved. (C-3)
47. _2_   I have no trouble solving problems involving other people.
48. _2_   I have trouble forgetting familiar things I should remember, such as my address, my telephone number, and names of close friends or family. (C-4)
49. _1_   I do not remember things as well as most people, such as names, what I did yesterday, or things in my past. (C-5)
50. _2_   I don't have any problems. (C-7)
51. _2_   I do not wish to make any changes in my life; I am happy the way things are. (C-6, C-7, C-8)
52. _4_   When I have a problem I would rather leave it unsolved than to spend a lot of time trying to solve it. (C-9)
53. _5_   I get mad if I spend too much time trying to solve a problem.
54. _3_   I have difficulty following directions. (C-10)
55. _4_   I do not like to follow directions given by other people.

Behavior (iii)

56. _5_   It seems I always do what others want to do rather than what I would like to do. (B-1)
57. _2_   During group discussion I find it hard to express my own views on a topic, especially when they differ from the views of other group members.
58. _1_   I have difficulty concentrating on one thing for very long. (B-2)
59. _2_   I never interrupt others during discussions. (B-3)
60. _2_   I make people mad by saying or doing the wrong things.
61. _2_   I find it difficult to look at the person to whom I am speaking. (B-4)
62. _5_   People get mad at me when I tell them what I want. (B-5)
63. _4_   I would rather others make decisions about major changes in my life. (B-6)
64. _5_   When people do something I don't like I may not cooperate with them (e.g., put things off they want me to do; be stubborn; half-heartedly participate in activities with them; not do as good a job for them as I would otherwise). (B-6)
65. _5_   I may yell at people and call them derogatory names (e.g., stupid, dumb) when they do something I don't like. (B-7)

66. _4_ I frequently lose my temper and argue with people.

67. _5_ I frequently lose my temper and hit people. (B-8)

Drugs (substance use or abuse, physical, and communication) (v)

68. _1_ I frequently drink excessively at home or at a bar. (D-1.1)

69. _1_ I take drugs during my leisure time.

70. _5_ I do not have a substance abuse problem (D-1.2)

71. _1_ I take drugs or drink alcohol to cope with my life stress and for relaxation. (D-1.3)

72. _4_ I do not exercise regularly. (D-2.1)

73. _4_ I bathe daily. (D-2.2)

74. _2_ I frequently experience one or more of the following: insomnia, lack of muscular endurance, awkwardness. (D-2.3 through D-2.7)

75. _1_ People have trouble understanding me when I speak. (D-3.1 through D-3.7)

Note for Examiner: Item numbers 4, 14, 16, 20, 43, 47, 59 and 73 should be scored by reversing the scale. These items are stated in the affirmative rather than in the negative. Item number 70 should be scored by reversing the scale if other assessments indicate the patient presently does not have a substance abuse problem.

PART III. POST INTERVIEW OBSERVATIONS

INSTRUCTIONS: Following termination of the above interview and dismissal of the examinee, the examiner should record the following post interview impressions using the scale below. Items requiring observation in music activities should be completed after observing the patient in music activities.

Strongly Inadequate	Inadequate	Mediocre	Adequate	Strongly Adequate
1	2	3	4	5

76. _2_ Rate the examinee's eye contact.

77. _4_ Rate the examinee's posture.

78. _3_ Rate the examinee's grooming.

79. _5_ Did the examinee appear motivated to engage in music therapy?

80. _3_ Did the examinee exhibit appropriate facial expressions?

81. _4_ Did the examinee engage in conversation, or what degree of conversational skill was observed?

82. _3_ How was the examinee's concentration?

83. _3_ How was the examinee's attention span?

84. _3_   How was the examinee's retention (e.g., Did test questions have to be repeated?)?

85. _2_   How well does the examinee use music (e.g., artistic, to reflect feelings or emotions, as an escape)?

86. _5_   Rate the examinee's overall attitude toward music.

87. _2_   Rate your initial impression of the quality of the examinee's overall interpersonal relationships.

88. _2_   How does the examinee perceive or solve problems during music activities?

89. _2_   Rate your initial impression of the examinee's overall level of self-concept.

90. _3_   Rate the examinee's abstracting ability (e.g., Did the examinee have trouble understanding the above questions? Did the examiner have to give a lot of examples?).

EXAMINER'S COMMENTS:

Construct a BASIC I.D. for Bob based on the above PMTQ results. You may refer to both the PMTQ items and the problems in this manual to which the PMTQ items are referenced. Remember that items rated a four or five (or one or two in the case of reversed scale items) are usually included in the BASIC I.D. as problems for possible intervention.

BASIC I.D.

MODALITY	PROBLEMS
Behavior	
Affect	
Sensation	
Imagery	
Cognitive	
Interpersonal	
Drugs	

Following completion of the above BASIC I.D., refer to the PMTQ results, the BASIC I.D., and the music therapy interventions in this manual to construct a Multimodal Music Therapy Profile.

Multimodal Music Therapy Profile: *D*

I. MUSIC PREFERENCES

_____

_____

_____

II. MULTIMODAL PROBLEM ANALYSIS

Interpersonal	Problem	Music Therapy Intervention
_____	_____	_____
_____	_____	_____
_____	_____	_____
_____	_____	_____

Affect	Problem	Music Therapy Intervention
_____	_____	_____
_____	_____	_____
_____	_____	_____

Cognitive	Problem	Music Therapy Intervention
_____	_____	_____
_____	_____	_____
_____	_____	_____

Behavior	Problem	Music Therapy Intervention
_____	_____	_____
_____	_____	_____
_____	_____	_____

Drugs	Problem	Music Therapy Intervention
_____	_____	_____
_____	_____	_____
_____	_____	_____

III. POST INTERVIEW OBSERVATIONS

_____

_____

Next, write one or more Music Therapy Intervention Plans for Bob.

MUSIC THERAPY INTERVENTION PLAN

NAME: _____   CASE NO: _____

DATE OF ASSESSMENT: _____

Music Therapy Goals and Objectives

Goal #__: _____

Goal Statement: _____

_____

Objective #__.__ Objective Statement:_____

_____

_____

Person Responsible: _____

Date Started: _____ Date Ended: _____

Reason Ended:_____

_____

Objective #__.__ Objective Statement:_____

_____

_____

Person Responsible: _____

Date Started: _____ Date Ended: _____

Reason Ended:_____

_____

Objective #__.__ Objective Statement:_____

_____

_____

Person Responsible: _____

Date Started: _____ Date Ended: _____

Reason Ended:_____

_____

Write one or more Implementation Strategies for Bob.

IMPLEMENTATION STRATEGY

NAME: _____   CASE NO: _____

DATE OF ASSESSMENT: _____

Objective #__.__: _____

_____

_____

Materials Needed: _____

_____

Reinforcement Schedule: _____

THERAPIST BEHAVIOR   PATIENT BEHAVIOR

_____   _____

_____   _____

_____   _____

_____   _____

_____   _____

_____   _____

_____   _____

_____   _____

_____   _____

_____   _____

_____   _____

_____   _____

_____   _____

_____   _____

_____   _____

_____   _____

_____   _____

_____   _____

_____   _____

Finally, write one or more Music Therapy Progress Report Charts for Bob. Be sure to write hypothetical progress reports for each session under Session Progress Report/Comments at the bottom of the chart.

Music Therapy Progress Report Chart

Name of Agency: _____

Patient Name: _____ Therapist Name: _____

Specify goal and objective being worked on in the space provided. Place the appropriate evaluation code under the session date to indicate whether or not the objective was met, if the patient or therapist was absent, or if there was insufficient time to work on the objective. Write a progress report for each session.

Goal #__: _____

_____

Objective #__.__: _____

_____

_____

Date: /   /   /   /   /   /

Progress:

EVALUATION:
Record a "+" for completion of objective.
Record a "P" for progress toward meeting the objective.
Record a "–" for not meeting objective.
Record an "A" for patient or therapist being absent
Record an "0" for insufficient time during the session to work on the objective.

Session Progress Report/Comments

_____

_____

_____

_____

_____

_____

_____

_____

_____

_____

_____

Adults: The case of James. Prior to his conviction on charges of child molestation of an adolescent male, James had successfully maintained employment as a city worker. After a brief imprisonment he was placed on parole and ordered to receive outpatient community mental health services. However, because of his previous conviction he was unable to obtain employment in the relatively small community in which he resided. Because of his fondness for music, James was subsequently referred to the music therapy clinic. From information in the following PMTQ, write a plan of treatment including a BASIC I.D., multimodal music therapy profile, intervention plan(s) and implementation strategy(ies), and hypothetical progress chart(s). To save space the clinical forms were omitted. Clinical forms for writing this treatment plan may be copied from Appendix IV.

PATIENT IDENTIFICATION FORM

NAME: James   SEX: Male   AGE: 40

DATE: July 15, 1997

FORMAL/PRIMARY DIAGNOSIS:

AXIS I: 302.20 Pedophilia, Sexually Attracted to Males, Exclusive

AXIS II: 301.82 Avoidant Personality Disorder

AXIS III: Stomach problems, vertigo

AXIS IV: Inadequate social support; living alone; unemployment; inadequate housing; inadequate finances; inadequate health insurance; incarceration.

AXIS V: Current GAF: 35   Highest GAF past year: 35

TOTAL NUMBER AND LENGTH OF STAYS OF PRIOR HOSPITALIZATIONS:

HOSPITAL	LENGTH OF STAY
One admission to the state hospital	30 days

LENGTH OF HOSPITALIZATION AT PRESENT FACILITY: Three years (in community placement and outpatient treatment).

TYPES OF MEDICATION TAKEN	*AND* DOSAGE PRESCRIBED
None	

PSYCHIATRIC MUSIC THERAPY QUESTIONNAIRE
ADULTS

INSTRUCTIONS: Parts I and II of the following questionnaire are to be administered by the **examiner, or therapist, interviewing the examinee, or patient.** Part III, Post Interview Observations, will be completed by the examiner following termination of the interview, or Part II.

EXAMINER: A major purpose of therapy is to assist you with problems that may be interfering with your ability to enjoy life to the fullest. The purpose of this questionnaire therefore, is to assist you in recognizing problems or "bad habits" you may have and wish to get rid of. Since these questions are personal, you may be assured of complete confidentiality. NO ONE WILL SEE YOUR ANSWERS OTHER THAN THE THERAPISTS. If you do not care to answer these questions simply tell me you do not care to answer these questions.

I. MUSIC (viii)

1. EXAMINER: For the following styles of music tell me the number that indicates the degree you like each type of music. (Examiner gives the attached scale, like the one below, to the examinee.)

	Strongly Dislike	Dislike	Neutral	Like	Strongly Like
COUNTRY	1	2	3	4	⑤
POPULAR	1	2	3	④	5
ROCK	1	2	3	④	5
JAZZ	1	2	3	4	⑤
FOLK	1	2	③	4	5
RELIGIOUS	1	2	3	④	5
OTHER: _____	1	2	3	4	5

2. EXAMINER: Who is your favorite performer or composer?
(INSTRUCTION: Examiner writes in name below)
Country: Hank Williams; Jazz: Louis Armstrong

INSTRUCTIONS FOR EXAMINER: Give the examinee the scale, like the one below, attached to this questionnaire. The examinee may then refer to the scale as necessary when choosing a number.

EXAMINER: I am going to read some statements. After each statement tell me the number from this scale that describes the extent you agree with the statement.

	Strongly Disagree	Disagree	Neutral	Agree	Strongly Agree
	1	2	3	4	5

3. _3_   I would like to participate in a group sing-a-long with a pianist or guitarist accompanying the group. (viii)

4. _2_   I would like to sing on stage before an audience.

5. _4_   I would like to learn to play a musical instrument.

II. MULTIMODAL PROBLEM ANALYSIS

INSTRUCTIONS FOR EXAMINER: Let the examinee continue to keep the scale, like the one below. The examinee may then refer to the scale as necessary when choosing a number.

EXAMINER: I am going to read some statements. After each statement tell me the number from this scale that describes the extent you agree with the statement.

	Strongly Disagree	Disagree	Neutral	Agree	Strongly Agree
	1	2	3	4	5

Interpersonal (iv)

1. _2_   I would rather be alone than be with people. (IS-1)

2. _4_   I find it hard to make friends.

3. _3_   I have no close friends.

4. _1_   It is easy for me to talk to people.

5. _4_   It is hard for me to talk when in a group of people.

6. _3_   I have trouble listening to others when they talk to me.

7. _2_   I do not have a hobby; I rarely do something just for fun. (IS-2, IS-4)

8. _3_   I would rather be alone or do nothing than to do something for fun with other people.

9. _3_   There is not much to do in my spare time other than to sleep or watch television.

10. _2_   I often get into trouble for not following directions, rules or regulations, or for not doing what I am suppose to do (e.g., smoking, eating, or drinking where prohibited). (IS-3)

11. _3_   Friendships or relationships with other people usually do not last more than one year. (IS-5)

12. _2_   I fight a lot with either my spouse (husband or wife) or family.

13. _4_ I would feel very uneasy telling a group of people my likes, dislikes, and personal experiences. (IS-6)

14. _2_ I have no difficulty being accepted by community groups (e.g., church, service groups) and with being invited to their events (e.g., parties, "get togethers"). (IS-7)

15. _3_ I would rather sit behind the group members or sit alone than to sit with the group. (IS-8)

16. _1_ I say the right things when trying to make friends with the opposite sex. (IS-9)

17. _3_ Listening to the problems of others is boring; I become impatient. (IS-10)

Affect (iii)

18. _4_ People cannot tell when I am happy, sad, or excited. (A-1)

19. _3_ I rarely feel happy, sad, excited, or smile.

20. _2_ I can easily tell when other people are happy, sad, or excited.

21. _2_ I never worry about anything. (A-2)

22. _3_ I never get angry or mad at people.

23. _2_ I frequently experience feelings of anger and stress (A-3)

24. _2_ I often hurt the feelings of my friends.

25. _2_ I often hit other people. (A-3, A-10)

26. _1_ I often feel like I have a tremendous amount of energy (i.e., difficulty sleeping, constantly moving and talking). (A-4)

27. _5_ I often feel like I have no energy and feel very sad. (A-5)

28. _3_ I frequently feel depressed or "down in the dumps."

29. _2_ I frequently feel like killing or hurting myself. (A-6)

30. _2_ I often wish I were dead.

31. _4_ I experience a lot of anxiety (A-7).

32. _4_ I often experience excessive anxiety from one or more of the following: present or past problems with other people, worry about the future (e.g., upcoming events), my life situation.

33. _4_ I often experience excessive anxiety that frequently results in one or more of the following: inability to relax, muscle stiffness, sleep disturbance, worry, verbally talking about my problems to myself or others.

34. _2_ It is easy for me to lose self-control and exhibit too much laughing, crying, or anger. (A-8)

35. _4_ I often become very, very scared along with one or more of the following: I get panicky, my heart beats fast, I experience shortness of breath. (A-9)

36. _2_ Sometimes I get so mad I could kill people. (A-10)

37. _2_ Sometimes I get so mad I hit people.

38. _3_ I frequently get mad when others give me advice.

39. _2_ People often tell me I have a bad temper.

Cognitive (iv)

40. _3_ I do not like myself. (C-1)
41. _3_ I frequently call myself names such as "stupid," "idiot," or "dumb."
42. _3_ I usually fail when I try to do something.
43. _4_ People like me.
44. _5_ I do not trust people. (C-2)
45. _4_ Other people frequently lie about me.
46. _3_ My problems are overwhelming; they can't be solved. (C-3)
47. _1_ I have no trouble solving problems involving other people.
48. _1_ I have trouble forgetting familiar things I should remember, such as my address, my telephone number, and names of close friends or family. (C-4)
49. _1_ I do not remember things as well as most people, such as names, what I did yesterday, or things in my past. (C-5)
50. _3_ I don't have any problems. (C-7)
51. _3_ I do not wish to make any changes in my life; I am happy the way things are. (C-6, C-7, C-8)
52. _4_ When I have a problem I would rather leave it unsolved than to spend a lot of time trying to solve it. (C-9)
53. _4_ I get mad if I spend too much time trying to solve a problem.
54. _5_ I have difficulty following directions. (C-10)
55. _5_ I do not like to follow directions given by other people.

Behavior (iii)

56. _4_ It seems I always do what others want to do rather than what I would like to do. (B-1)
57. _3_ During group discussion I find it hard to express my own views on a topic, especially when they differ from the views of other group members.
58. _4_ I have difficulty concentrating on one thing for very long. (B-2)
59. _3_ I never interrupt others during discussions. (B-3)
60. _3_ I make people mad by saying or doing the wrong things.
61. _4_ I find it difficult to look at the person to whom I am speaking. (B-4)
62. _2_ People get mad at me when I tell them what I want. (B-5)
63. _2_ I would rather others make decisions about major changes in my life. (B-6)
64. _4_ When people do something I don't like I may not cooperate with them (e.g., put things off they want me to do; be stubborn; half-heartedly participate in activities with them; not do as good a job for them as I would otherwise). (B-6)
65. _1_ I may yell at people and call them derogatory names (e.g., stupid, dumb) when they do something I don't like. (B-7)

66. _2_ I frequently lose my temper and argue with people.

67. _1_ I frequently lose my temper and hit people. (B-8)

Drugs (substance use or abuse, physical, and communication) (v)

68. _3_ I frequently drink excessively at home or at a bar. (D-1.1)

69. _1_ I take drugs during my leisure time.

70. _2_ I do not have a substance abuse problem (D-1.2)

71. _3_ I take drugs or drink alcohol to cope with my life stress and for relaxation. (D-1.3)

72. _5_ I do not exercise regularly. (D-2.1)

73. _2_ I bathe daily. (D-2.2)

74. _5_ I frequently experience one or more of the following: insomnia, lack of muscular endurance, awkwardness. (D-2.3 through D-2.7)

75. _4_ People have trouble understanding me when I speak. (D-3.1 through D-3.7)

Note for Examiner: Item numbers 4, 14, 16, 20, 43, 47, 59 and 73 should be scored by reversing the scale. These items are stated in the affirmative rather than in the negative. Item number 70 should be scored by reversing the scale if other assessments indicate the patient presently does not have a substance abuse problem.

PART III. POST INTERVIEW OBSERVATIONS

INSTRUCTIONS: Following termination of the above interview and dismissal of the examinee, the examiner should record the following post interview impressions using the scale below. Items requiring observation in music activities should be completed after observing the patient in music activities.

Strongly Inadequate	Inadequate	Mediocre	Adequate	Strongly Adequate
1	2	3	4	5

76. _3_ Rate the examinee's eye contact.

77. _2_ Rate the examinee's posture.

78. _2_ Rate the examinee's grooming.

79. _4_ Did the examinee appear motivated to engage in music therapy?

80. _3_ Did the examinee exhibit appropriate facial expressions?

81. _3_ Did the examinee engage in conversation, or what degree of conversational skill was observed?

82. _3_ How was the examinee's concentration?

83. _3_ How was the examinee's attention span?

84. _2_ How was the examinee's retention (e.g., Did test questions have to be repeated?)?

85. _4_ How well does the examinee use music (e.g., artistic, to reflect feelings or emotions, as an escape)?

86. _5_ Rate the examinee's overall attitude toward music.

87. _3_ Rate your initial impression of the quality of the examinee's overall interpersonal relationships.

88. _3_ How does the examinee perceive or solve problems during music activities?

89. _2_ Rate your initial impression of the examinee's overall level of self-concept.

90. _3_ Rate the examinee's abstracting ability (e.g., Did the examinee have trouble understanding the above questions? Did the examiner have to give a lot of examples?).

EXAMINER'S COMMENTS:

Adolescents: The case of Kathy. Kathy was receiving residential care from a community mental health center upon her referral to the music therapy clinic. From information in the following PMTQ, write a plan of treatment for Kathy including a BASIC I.D., multimodal music therapy profile, intervention plan(s), implementation strategy(ies), and hypothetical progress chart(s). Clinical forms for writing this treatment plan may be copied from Appendix IV.

PATIENT IDENTIFICATION FORM

NAME: Kathy _____ SEX: Female __ AGE: 16 _____

DATE: August 12, 1998 _____

FORMAL/PRIMARY DIAGNOSIS: (unknown)

AXIS I: _____

AXIS II: _____

AXIS III: _____

AXIS IV: _____

AXIS V: Current GAF: _____ Highest GAF past year: _____

TOTAL NUMBER AND LENGTH OF STAYS OF PRIOR HOSPITALIZATIONS:

HOSPITAL	LENGTH OF STAY
Unknown	Unknown

LENGTH OF HOSPITALIZATION AT PRESENT FACILITY: Six weeks _____

TYPES OF MEDICATION TAKEN	*AND* DOSAGE PRESCRIBED
None	

PSYCHIATRIC MUSIC THERAPY QUESTIONNAIRE
ADOLESCENTS

INSTRUCTIONS: Parts I and II of the following questionnaire are to be administered by the **examiner, or therapist, interviewing the examinee, or patient.** Part III, Post Interview Observations, will be completed by the examiner following termination of the interview, or Part II.

EXAMINER: A major purpose of therapy is to assist you with problems that may be interfering with your ability to enjoy life to the fullest. The purpose of this questionnaire therefore, is to assist you in recognizing problems or "bad habits" you may have and wish to get rid of. Since these questions are personal, you may be assured of complete confidentiality. NO ONE WILL SEE YOUR ANSWERS OTHER THAN THE THERAPISTS. If you do not care to answer these questions simply tell me you do not care to answer these questions.

I. MUSIC (x)

1. EXAMINER: For the following styles of music tell me the number that indicates the degree you like each type of music. (Examiner shows the following scale to the examinee).

	Strongly Dislike	Dislike	Neutral	Like	Strongly Like
COUNTRY	1	2	③	4	5
POPULAR	①	2	3	4	5
ROCK	①	2	3	4	5
JAZZ	1	2	3	④	5
FOLK	①	2	3	4	5
RELIGIOUS	1	2	3	④	5
OTHER: *Rap*	1	2	3	4	⑤

2. EXAMINER: Who is your favorite performer or composer?
(INSTRUCTION: Examiner writes in name below)
Does not have one.

INSTRUCTIONS FOR EXAMINER: Give the examinee the scale, like the one below, attached to this questionnaire. The examinee may then refer to the scale as necessary when choosing a number.

EXAMINER: I am going to read some statements. After each statement tell me the number from this scale that describes the extent you agree with the statement.

	Strongly Disagree	Disagree	Neutral	Agree	Strongly Agree
	1	2	3	4	5

3. _4_ I would like to learn to play a musical instrument. (x)
4. _4_ I would like to play a musical instrument for others.
5. _5_ I would probably enjoy playing a musical instrument if I knew how (improvisation).
6. _1_ I would like to participate in a group sing-a-long with a pianist or guitarist accompanying the group.
7. _5_ I would like to learn to write music. *Especially Rap*

II. MULTIMODAL PROBLEM ANALYSIS

INSTRUCTIONS FOR EXAMINER: Let the examinee continue to keep the scale, like the one below. The examinee may then refer to the scale as necessary when choosing a number.

EXAMINER: I am going to read some statements. After each statement tell me the number from this scale that describes the extent you agree with the statement.

	Strongly Disagree	Disagree	Neutral	Agree	Strongly Agree
	1	2	3	4	5

Affect (vi)
1. _3_ Other people know when I am happy, sad, or excited. (A-1)
2. _2_ I rarely feel happy, sad, or excited.
3. _5_ I can easily tell when other people are happy, sad, or excited.
4. _4_ I often hurt the feelings of my friends. (A-2)
5. _5_ I often hit other people.
6. _5_ I often get mad at others.
7. _1_ I often get mad at myself.
8. _4_ I often hurt or feel like hurting myself.
9. _1_ I often feel like destroying things that others have.
10. _1_ I don't fight with or yell at others.
11. _4_ I often feel like I am under a lot of stress. (A-3)
12. _5_ Because of stress, I often experience one or more of the following: trouble sleeping, stomach aches, anxiety, and/or doing things I later regret.

13. _4_   I experience a lot of anxiety. (A-4)

14. _5_   My excessive anxiety frequently results from one or more of the following: present or past problems with other people; worry about the future (e.g., upcoming events).

15. _5_   I frequently do things I later am sorry for. (A-5)

16. _5_   It is hard for me to tell other people about bad things that happen to me. (A-6)

17. _1_   It is hard for me to tell other people about good things that happen to me.

18. _4_   I frequently feel depressed or "down in the dumps." (A-7)

19. _1_   I frequently feel like killing myself. (A-8)

20. _4_   It is easy to say nice things to people. (A-9)

Interpersonal (vi)

21. _5_   I rarely get into trouble for not following rules and regulations, or not doing what I am suppose to do. (IS-1)

22. _2_   I have trouble following directions (e.g., Stay in your chair; Finish your work; Work quietly; Be nice to others).

23. _5_   I like to take turns and to share my things with others.

24. _1_   I frequently get into trouble on and off hospital/school grounds.

25. _5_   I like to tell others when they make a mistake. (IS-2)

26. _3_   I frequently call people names such as "stupid," "idiot," or "dumb."

27. _2_   I would rather be alone than be with people. (IS-3)

28. _5_   I find it hard to make friends.

29. _4_   I have no close friends.

30. _2_   It is hard for me to talk to people.

31. _2_   It is hard for me to talk when in a group of people.

32. _1_   I spend most of my leisure time with a gang or in a bar. (IS-4)

33. _1_   I do not have a hobby; I rarely do something just for fun (IS-4 through IS-5)

34. _1_   I would rather be alone or do nothing than to do something with other people. (IS-5 through IS-6)

35. _2_   I have trouble listening to others when they talk to me. (IS-6)

Cognitive (vi)

36. _1_   I do not like myself. (C-1)

37. _1_   I frequently call myself names such as "stupid," "idiot," or "dumb."

38. _2_   I usually fail when I try to do something.

39. _3_   People do not like me.

40. _1_ I have a lot of problems. (C-2)
41. _5_ I have no trouble solving problems involving other people.
42. _5_ When I have a problem I would rather leave it unsolved than to spend a lot of time trying to solve it. (C-3)
43. _3_ I get mad if I spend too much time trying to solve a problem.
44. _3_ I do not trust other people. (C-4)
45. _5_ Other people frequently lie about me.
46. _1_ It bothers me for someone to tell me how I could do something better. (C-5)
47. _1_ I never have any problems. (C-6)
48. _2_ I have trouble keeping track of things; I frequently lose things (e.g., bills, records, money). (C-7)
49. _1_ I am always fighting with my parents. (C-8 through C-10)
50. _5_ I have no trouble making decisions (e.g., What I would like to do each day, what to eat for dinner, where to go, what music to listen to, what clothes to wear). (C-13)

Drugs (substance use or abuse) (vii)

51. _1_ Drugs will not hurt me psychologically or physically. (D-1.1)
52. _1_ I take drugs regularly. (D-1.1 through D-1.2)
53. _5_ I do not have a substance abuse problem. (D-1.2)
54. _1_ I take drugs or drink alcohol to cope with my life stress, unpleasant situations, or to block unpleasant feelings. (D-1.2)

Behavior (vi)

55. _4_ It seems I always do what others want to do rather than what I would like to do. (B-1)
56. _4_ During group discussion I find it hard to express my own views on a topic, especially when they differ from the views of other group members.
57. _5_ I have difficulty concentrating on, or doing one thing for very long. (B-2, B-5)
58. _5_ I usually leave or keep to myself when in a group. (B-3)

Note for Examiner: Item numbers 1, 3, 10, 20, 21, 23, 41, and 50 should be scored by reversing the scale. These items are stated in the affirmative rather than in the negative. Item number 53 should be scored by reversing the scale if other assessments indicate the patient presently does not have a substance abuse problem.

PART III. POST INTERVIEW OBSERVATIONS

INSTRUCTIONS: Following termination of the above interview and dismissal of the examinee, the examiner should record the following post interview impressions using the scale below.

Strongly Inadequate	Inadequate	Mediocre	Adequate	Strongly Adequate
1	2	3	.4	5

59. _5_ Rate your initial impression of the quality of examinee's overall interpersonal relationships.

60. _3_ How well does the examinee use music (e.g., artistic; to reflect feelings or emotions; as an escape)?

61. _5_ How does the examinee perceive, perpetuate, or solve problems during music activities?

62. _5_ How was the examinee's concentration?

63. _5_ How was the examinee's attention span?

64. _4_ How was the examinee's retention (e.g., Did test questions have to be repeated?)?

65. _4_ Rate the examinee's eye contact.

66. _5_ Rate the examinee's posture.

67. _5_ Rate the examinee's grooming.

68. _4_ Did the examinee appear motivated to engage in music therapy?

69. _4_ Did the examinee exhibit appropriate facial expressions?

70. _4_ Did the examinee engage in conversation, or what degree of conversational skill was observed?

71. _5_ Rate your initial impression of the examinee's overall level of self-concept.

72. _5_ Rate the examinee's musical creativity or ability.

73. _5_ Rate the examinee's overall attitude toward music.

EXAMINER'S COMMENTS:

Childhood: The case of Allen. Allen was receiving play therapy and music therapy at the local mental health center. The following PMTQ was administered to Allen's mother as part of Allen's music therapy assessment. From information in the following PMTQ, write a plan of treatment including a BASIC I.D., multimodal music therapy profile(s), intervention plan(s) and implementation strategy(ies), and hypothetical progress chart(s). To save space the clinical forms were omitted. Clinical forms for writing this treatment plan may be copied from Appendix IV.

PATIENT IDENTIFICATION FORM

NAME: Allen   SEX: Male   AGE: 7

DATE: May 11, 1998

FORMAL/PRIMARY DIAGNOSIS:

AXIS I: PTSD (Post Traumatic Stress Syndrome), Acute

ADHD (Attention-Deficit-Hyperactivity Disorder) NOS

Pervasive Developmental Disorder NOS

AXIS II: None

AXIS III: Premature birth at 32 weeks

AXIS IV: Sexual abuse; Removal from the home

AXIS V: Current GAF: 55   Highest GAF past year: 60

TOTAL NUMBER AND LENGTH OF STAYS OF PRIOR HOSPITALIZATIONS: NA

HOSPITAL   LENGTH OF STAY

LENGTH OF HOSPITALIZATION AT PRESENT FACILITY: Four weeks

TYPES OF MEDICATION TAKEN   *AND* DOSAGE PRESCRIBED

Dexedrine   25 mg daily

Clonidine   .05 mg 2 times daily

PSYCHIATRIC MUSIC THERAPY QUESTIONNAIRE
CHILDREN

INSTRUCTIONS FOR EXAMINER: Parts I and II of the following questionnaire are to be administered by the examiner, or therapist, **interviewing a second person (examinee) who is familiar with the child**. The examinee is to be dismissed after finishing Part II.

EXAMINER: A major purpose of therapy is to assist persons with problems that may be interfering with their ability to experience success in life. The purpose of this questionnaire therefore, is to assist you in recognizing your child's problems or inappropriate behavior that you would like to see changed. Since these questions are personal, you may be assured of complete confidentiality. NO ONE WILL SEE YOUR ANSWERS OTHER THAN THE THERAPISTS. If you do not care to answer these questions simply tell me you do not care to answer these questions.

I. MUSIC (xi)

1. INSTRUCTION: Examiner gives the attached music preference scale to the examinee.

EXAMINER: For the following styles of music tell me the number that indicates the degree [PATIENT'S NAME] likes each type of music.

	Strongly Dislike	Dislike	Neutral	Like	Strongly Like
COUNTRY	①	2	3	4	5
POPULAR	1	2	3	4	⑤
ROCK	①	2	3	4	5
CHILDREN'S	①	2	3	4	5
FOLK	①	2	3	4	5
RELIGIOUS	①	2	3	4	5
OTHER: *Rap*	1	2	3	4	⑤

2. EXAMINER: Can you tell me [PATIENT'S NAME]'s favorite recording, performer, or composer? (INSTRUCTION: Examiner writes in name below)

Does not have a favorite performer or composer.

INSTRUCTIONS FOR EXAMINER: Give the examinee the scale, like the one below, attached to this questionnaire. The examinee may then refer to the scale as necessary when choosing a number.

EXAMINER: I am going to read some statements. After each statement tell me the number from this scale that describes the extent the statement describes [PATIENT'S NAME].

	Strongly Disagree	Disagree	Neutral	Agree	Strongly Agree
	1	2	3	4	5

3. _3_ Is able to identify characteristics of music such as style, slow or fast, which instruments are playing, and whether an instrument is playing or a person is singing. (xi)

4. _4_ Sings melody in tune. (xi)

5. _1_ Would enjoy playing a musical instrument. (xi)

6. _4_ Would enjoy making up own movements to music. (xi)

II. MULTIMODAL PROBLEM ANALYSIS

INSTRUCTIONS FOR EXAMINER: Let the examinee continue to keep the scale, like the one below. The examinee may then refer to the scale as necessary when choosing a number.

EXAMINER: I am going to read some statements. After each statement tell me the number from this scale that describes the extent the statement describes [PATIENT'S NAME].

	Strongly Disagree	Disagree	Neutral	Agree	Strongly Agree
	1	2	3	4	5

Interpersonal (vii)

1. _5_ Rarely gets into trouble for not following rules and regulations, or not doing what he/she is suppose to do. (IS-1)

2. _5_ Has trouble following directions (e.g., Stay in your chair; Finish your work; Work quietly; Be nice to others).

3. _4_ Exhibits disruptive outbursts such as temper tantrums to attract attention.

4. _4_ Is liked by peers.

5. _5_ Frequently calls others names such as "stupid," "idiot," or "dumb."

6. _2_ Does not talk, or talks very little with peers. (IS-2)

7. _2_ Does not participate or avoids participating in group activities with peers.

8. _1_ Is shy, timid, and not interested in peers.

9. _5_ Argues with peers. (IS-3)

10. _4_ Does not cooperate when working or playing with peers.

11. _2_ Likes to take turns and to share things with others. (IS-4)

12. _5_ Does not pay attention to others while participating in structured activities. (IS-5)

13. __1__ Speaks too softly to be heard by others. (IS-6)

14. __1__ Demonstrates good leadership skills (e.g., team captain). (IS-7)

15. __4__ Does not express or respond to greetings or closings (e.g., good-byes, hellos). (IS-8)

Behavior (vii)

16. __2__ Does not express needs or wants to others. (B-1)

17. __2__ Goes along with the group instead of stating own opinions or feelings.

18. __5__ Does not stay on task, is too easily distracted, and has poor concentration. (B-2)

19. __5__ Grabs things from others instead of sharing or taking turns. (B-3)

20. __5__ Hits peers. (B-4)

21. __5__ Has poor eye contact; does not look at person speaking, or when speaking; looks away or down when speaking or being spoken to. (B-5)

Drugs (Motor) (viii)

22. __1__ Awkward when attempting common movements such as walking. (D-1.1)

23. __2__ Runs into people when in a group.

24. __2__ Cannot use fingers to perform tasks as well as peers (e.g., picking up coins, grasping a pencil, dialing a telephone number, turning pages of a book [finger dexterity]). (D-1.2 through D-1.3)

25. __4__ Catches ball, claps hands, hits toy drum with ease. (D-1.4)

26. __2__ Often drops objects causing disruptions to others and embarrassment to self. (D-1.5)

27. __2__ Cannot recall recent family events such as a trip to the park. (D-2.1)

28. __4__ Has trouble imitating speech or sounds. (D-2.2)

29. __4__ Talks too loud. (D-2.3)

30. __5__ Does not pronounce words clearly. (D-2.4)

31 __4__ Has trouble comprehending what is said to him or her. (D-2.5)

Cognitive (vii)

32. __5__ Has trouble with following directions. (C-1)

33. __1__ Understands concepts such as left and right, behind, in front of, and next to, or over, under, around, and through. (C-2)

34. __5__ Makes negative comments about self, such as "I'm dumb" or "I'm not very smart." (C-3)

35. __4__ Refuses to participate in group or individual activities because of a lack of self-confidence (e.g., afraid of failure or ridicule). (C-3)

36. _5_ Exhibits one or more of the following when performing tasks: disorganized rather than goal directed; fast without concern for quality rather than slow and deliberate; gives up easily rather than demonstrating perseverance; inaccurate rather than accurate. (C-4)

37. _5_ Makes derogatory comments to peers if they don't do what he or she wants. (C-5)

38. _5_ Has trouble telling what time it is, or the day of the week. (C-6)

39. _2_ Has trouble counting money. (C-7)

40. _1_ Has trouble memorizing the letters of the alphabet. (C-8)

41. _2_ Has trouble counting. (C-9)

Affect (vii)

42. _5_ Other people know when he or she is happy, sad, or excited. (A-1)

43. _1_ Shows little or no emotion (e.g., happy, sad, or excited).

44. _2_ Can easily tell when other people are happy, sad, or excited.

45. _4_ Has trouble describing how others feel.

46. _4_ Exhibits too many emotional extremes (e.g., laughing or crying, happy or sad).

47. _2_ Emotions which are exhibited are frequently inappropriate for the occasion or situation (e.g., laughs in sad situations or when sad, cries when happy or in happy situations).

Note for Examiner: The above item numbers 1, 4, 11, 14, 25, 33, 42, and 44 should be scored by reversing the scale. These items are stated in the affirmative rather than in the negative.

PART III. POST INTERVIEW OBSERVATIONS

INSTRUCTIONS FOR THE EXAMINER: Part III, Post Interview Observations, is to be completed by the music therapist after observing the patient in music therapy. Rate items 48 through 62 using the following scale.

Strongly Inadequate	Inadequate	Mediocre	Adequate	Strongly Adequate
1	2	3	4	5

48. _3_ Concentration

49. _3_ Attention span

50. _2_ Retention

51. _3_ Interpersonal relationships

52. _2_ Eye contact

53. _4_ Posture

54. _4_ Grooming

55. _3_ Motivation to engage in music therapy

56. _4_ Appropriate facial expressions

57. _3_ Engages in conversation; degree of conversational skill

58. _2_ Perceives and solves problems during music activities

59. _3_ Uses music appropriately (e.g., artistic, to reflect feelings or emotions, as an escape)

60. _4_ Musical creativity or ability

61. _3_ Overall attitude toward music

62. _5_ Rhythmic ability

63. Does the patient have any handicapping conditions that may impair activity participation?

YES   (CIRCLE ONE)

(If YES, explain below under COMMENTS)

EXAMINER'S COMMENTS:

CHAPTER 10

GROUP THERAPY

G roup therapy is the mode of treatment in many psychiatric facilities usually because of a lack of man power and funding that would be required for one-to-one therapy. Most schools of psychotherapy that originated as one-to-one therapy have been adapted for group therapy. Group therapy however, has numerous advantages, and is not considered a second rate choice to one-to-one therapy. One psychiatrist treating substance abuse patients stated he preferred group therapy because if 12 patients told a patient he or she was mistaken, it would be more effective than if he alone told the patient. Weiten and Lloyd (1994) have noted three major advantages of group therapy. One major advantage is that patients realize their problems are not unique. They frequently observe patients with worse problems and greater misery than their own. Another advantage is that group therapy provides a safe setting in which to practice interpersonal skills. In a large sense, lack of interpersonal skills, or the inability to get along with others is the primary reason persons seek therapy. Group therapy is considered far superior to one-to-one therapy for the development of interpersonal skills. A third advantage of group therapy is that certain types of problems are especially well suited for group therapy. Some people respond especially well to group therapy because it provides them with mutual support from others with similar problems as they work on their own problems. There are many peer self-help groups in which people get together for mutual support such as former psychiatric patients and Alcoholics Anonymous.

The use of music in group therapy has long been advocated and practiced in the music therapy profession (Gaston, 1968). Guidelines have been published for the use of music in group therapy (Plach, 1980), books exist describing group activities for use in music therapy (Schulberg, 1981) and that describe music group therapy procedures (Plach, 1980; Unkefer, 1990; Wolfe, Burns, Stoll, & Wichmann, 1975), and research exists documenting the clinical usage and effects of music group therapy (Cassity, 1994; 1995; Cassity & Theobold, 1990; Ficken, 1976; Rubin, 1976; Thaut, 1994).

As indicated in Chapter 1, multimodal therapy may be conducted as group therapy. The use of music may make multimodal therapy even more amenable to group therapy. Rather than addressing one problem at a time, a music therapy intervention can simultaneously address a variety of problems across numerous modalities and individuals. For example, a rock band was one group therapy intervention used with Scott, David, John, and Ron who were residing at an adolescent detention center. During a rehearsal, John exhibited greater frustration tolerance at problem solving while learning to play the piano part (Cognitive), Scott who distanced others through excessively negative and uncooperative behavior had to listen to others and blend his playing in with the playing of others as he played the trap drum set (Interpersonal), David who had a history of withdrawal and nonverbalization in groups served as the group's vocalist and participated in critiques of the group performance (Interpersonal), and Ron who had low self-esteem, a lack of self-confidence, and inappropriate leisure skills learned the socially valued skill of playing the electric guitar.

Procedure

Although more than one method exists for practicing group therapy (Weiten & Lloyd, 1994), we have found the following procedure to be a viable one for routine use in group therapy with adults and adolescents. It is recommended that the reader study Chapters 2 and 9 before attempting to understand the information in this chapter. The following group therapy examples are presented with the open acknowledgment that they may not generalize or be applicable in all group music therapy situations. One example we use involves a group of adolescents who were admitted as a group for a six week stay at a residential facility. They therefore participated in their total treatment program, including music therapy, as a group for six weeks. It is recognized that other group music therapy situations may differ, such as a situation in which patients are continuously admitted and discharged from an ongoing music therapy group. The purpose of the following paragraphs however, is to report our experiences at using multimodal group music therapy. Like multimodal music therapy in general, we have found the group model to be quiet flexible and believe it can be adapted to a variety of music therapy situations. In addition, because of confidentiality restraints, all adolescents referred to in this chapter are a composite of the many adolescent patients with whom the authors have worked. Since these adolescents represent *typical* adolescent patients, any resemblance to real or actual persons is purely coincidental.

During the first session the patients are greeted, and name tags may be used to assist the therapists and patients with learning one another's names. Following the initial greeting, we attempt to give the group a sense of direction and expectation by informing them about music therapy, the benefits of group music therapy, and the types of activities they will be participating in. The patients are then administered the PMTQ. Following administration of the PMTQ, if time and confidentiality permits, we find it usually increases patient motivation to let them observe a live or video taped presentation of senior or past patients modeling the types of activities planned. We also demonstrate the instruments and any nontraditional techniques we will use. Each subsequent session is begun with a greeting, followed by an explanation of the goals for the session, and a description of the activities that are planned.

Following the initial session, the general procedure for planning group therapy experiences is to (1) examine each patient's PMTQ to determine problems the patient has in common with the other group members and/or problems amenable to treatment in group therapy, (2) formulate a Group BASIC I.D. containing problems derived in step one, and (3) write an individualized multimodal treatment plan on each client that is based on the Group BASIC I.D.

Examining each patient's PMTQ. If more than one therapist is working with the group we usually find it most efficient to have the therapists meet in a "staffing" to discuss the results of each patient's PMTQ to determine problems the patients have in common. Any ancillary assessment information from the patients themselves or their staff also is considered. Before arriving to the staffing each therapist constructs an individualized BASIC I.D. on his or her assigned patient so that individual needs may be considered when formulating the Group BASIC I.D. Also the therapists may decide whether the group is appropriate for treating the unique problems of a given patient. The staffing terminates with the construction of a Group BASIC I.D., an agreement on which problems are to be treated first, and the types of music therapy activities to be used. The group therapy plan is then presented to the patients at the following music therapy session for their endorsement.

If upon occasion a patient needs individualized therapy, then such therapy usually is provided in conjunction with group therapy. For example, Charles, age 16, diagnosed with attention deficit disorder and dyslexia, and was placed by the court in a residential facility because of a conviction stemming from the possession of marijuana. The initial music therapy assessment revealed his high degree of past failure probably was responsible for his low self-esteem, low frustration tolerance, and deteriorating interpersonal relationships. Charles also indicated he once played the piano and expressed a desire to resume piano lessons. It therefore was decided for Charles to resume piano lessons as individualized therapy with the goals of increasing his self-esteem and self-confidence through a successful experience, increasing frustration tolerance for problem solving, and developing a leisure skill (before his court commitment he spent his leisure time in a bar or with gang members). In addition to one-to-one therapy, Charles also was involved in group music therapy to treat his interpersonal problems as well as other problems that were common to the members of his group.

Formulating a Group BASIC I.D.

Following is an example of a Group BASIC I.D. constructed for a group of six male and two female adolescents receiving treatment at an adolescent detention center. Music therapy sessions were held for one hour once a week. The adolescents, in terms of diagnosis and GAF, were typical of the types of adolescents music therapists most frequently treat (Appendix I; Cassity & Cassity, 1994).

GROUP BASIC I.D.

MODALITY	PROBLEMS	
Behavior	B-1:	Lack of assertiveness – Kathy
	B-2:	Lacks attention to task – Kathy
	B-3:	Withdraws or isolates self in social situations – Kathy
Affect	A-1:	Inability to identify/express feelings – Austin, Alan, Ted, Skip, Melanie
	A-2:	Exhibits anger toward others – Alan, James, Bob, Skip, Kathy
		Indicates anger toward self – Melanie; Kathy
	A-3:	Experiences stress reactions – Alan, Austin, Bob, Kathy
	A-5:	Lacks self-control; poor impulse control – Alan, Skip, Kathy
	A-6:	Difficulty sharing own feelings with others – Melanie, Kathy
Sensation	NA	
Imagery	NA	
Cognitive	C-1:	Low self-esteem – Alan
	C-2:	Lacks problem solving skills – Alan, Austin
	C-3:	Gives up easily when solving problems; low frustration tolerance – Alan, James, Kathy
	C-4:	Does not trust others – Melanie, Kathy
Interpersonal	IS-1:	Uncooperative behavior; does not follow directions – Alan, James, Austin, Bob, Skip
	IS-2:	Lacks awareness of self or others – Alan, Ted, Bob (name calling); Melanie, Kathy (Overly critical of others)
	IS-4:	Inappropriate use of leisure time – Alan, James, Austin, Skip
Drugs	D-1.1:	Unaware of or denies chemical dependency or loss of self-control; may lack knowledge of the effects of chemicals upon physical and psychological functioning – Alan, James, Skip?
	D-1.2:	Uses substances regularly – Alan, James, Skip?

Each group music therapy session was divided into two 30 minute segments. During the first 30 minutes the type of music therapy intervention presented varied from week to week and was designed to address specific patient problems. During the second 30 minutes the patients rehearsed in the patient rock band consisting of electronic keyboard, trap drums and other percussion, electric guitar, and vocals. This second intervention was chosen because of its reinforcement potential and therapeutic value to the adolescents being treated.

The adolescents followed by their chronological ages were Ted, 18; Kathy, 18; James, 16; Melanie, 15; Austin, 15; Skip, 15; Bob, 14; and Alan, 13. A perusal of the above Group BASIC I.D. indicates interpersonal, cognitive, affective, and behavioral deficits, with numerous specific problems common to at least half of the group members. Of the eight patients, six revealed interpersonal problems of lack of awareness of self or others, five indicated uncooperative behavior/not following directions, and four inappropriately used their leisure time (e.g., no hobbies; spends time in a bar or with a gang). At least half the group members also had affective problems. Six indicated anger towards others or self, and five indicated the inability to identify/express feelings.

Also indicated in the above Group BASIC I.D., James strongly agreed he takes drugs regularly and that he does not have a substance abuse problem. Alan simply agreed with the two statements. A question mark is entered after Skip's name since he neither agreed nor disagreed (neutral) with the PMTQ statements that "Drugs will not hurt me psychologically or physically" and "I take drugs or drink alcohol to cope with my life stress, unpleasant situations, or to block unpleasant feelings." The remaining five patients, Ted, Kathy, Melanie, Austin, and Bob, were against substance use or abuse. Based on the above information it was decided to include substance abuse in the Group BASIC I.D. It was also decided to have a music therapy intervention during the first 30 minutes of the next session focusing on lyric analysis and discussion of a song illustrating the hazards of substance abuse. It is interesting to note that two of the three patients who indicated they were against substance abuse made positive contributions in the follow-up music therapy session. When discussing a topic that may be highly threatening such as the above, it may be advisable to use systematic desensitization to provide for a less threatening approach. For example, the therapist might first discuss the music characteristics of the song, then the message of the lyrics, then the consequences of drug abuse followed by individualized substance abuse problems of the group members, and finally rehabilitative concerns such as alternative turn-ons and other changes in life-style. Activities such as the above, conducted during the initial 30 minutes of the session, were by nature more verbal, whereas the rock band activity conducted during the final 30 minutes was more of a nonverbal therapeutic approach.

The Group Basic I.D. also indicates Kathy and Alan had problems apparently not shared by the other group members. Kathy was the only group member with the Behavioral problems lack of assertiveness, lack of attention to task and withdrawal or isolation in social situations. These problems were indicated in Kathy's PMTQ interview in which she indicated she has difficulty expressing her views in a group, difficulty concentrating on one thing for very long, and that she usually leaves or keeps to herself when in a group. These problems were probably related to other less common problems Kathy shared with Melanie, such as difficulty sharing own feelings with others (A-6), and lack of trust of others (C-4). Alan was the only patient who indicated low self-esteem. The PMTQ analysis indicated Alan frequently thought of himself in derogatory terms, stated he usually fails, and indicated people do not like him. Although some of Kathy and Alan's problems were not shared by the other group members, it was decided that such unique problems could also be treated in group music therapy along with problems the patients had in common.

As previously indicated, the rock band was used as a music therapy intervention the second 30 minutes of the session. Because the therapy was time limited (six weeks), nontraditional guitar (EZ Chord) and piano techniques were used to provide for immediate reinforcement. Success in the rock band was contingent upon following directions, cooperation, self and other awareness, frustration tolerance in problem solving situations, self-control, and impulse control. In addition the patients had the opportunity to develop a socially valued leisure skill. Kathy worked on her problems on both a nonverbal and verbal level as a vocalist for the band (nonverbal) and by making constructive comments about the performances (verbal). Her role as vocalist led to greater assertiveness, attention to task, presence in the group, and increased positive comments toward others. The acceptance and recognition Alan got from his contributions to the band increased his self-esteem as evidenced by a decrease in the number of self-deprecating statements. Although many problems on the above Group BASIC I.D. could be treated in either the first or second half of the session, the rock band appeared more effective at breaking through resistances of the hardest to reach patients. This may have been because of the nature of the activity which, aside from its reinforcement value, was more nonverbal and perhaps less threatening than activities such as lyric analysis.

Writing an individualized multimodal treatment plan on each client that is based on the Group BASIC I.D. Once the Group BASIC I.D. has been constructed each patient's individualized treatment plan is constructed, based on the Group BASIC I.D. The format of the treatment plan is the same as described in Chapter 2, consisting of the Multimodal Music Therapy Profile, Music Therapy intervention Plans, Implementation Strategies, and Music Therapy Progress Report Charts. Although the above procedure is focused on determining problems the group has in common, this should not be the overriding concern. Top priority should be assigned to meeting the needs of each patient. As indicated previously, the patient may have problems that require one-to-one therapy, or have unique problems that could be treated in group therapy despite their dissimilarity to the problems of the other group members.

Although it is still a matter of debate as to whether it is best to have a homogeneous group (e.g., similar problems, sex and age) for group therapy (Weiten & Lloyd, 1994), we usually take a "middle of the road" approach to this controversy. While selecting problems the group has in common may increase group cohesiveness, motivation and interest among group members, it also is important to remember that a problem need not be shared by all group members for it to be included in the Group BASIC I.D. The problems in the above Group BASIC I.D. were shared by some of the group, but not all of the group. It may even be counterproductive if patients all have the same problem if they do not believe they need treatment for the problem. In the above substance abuse example, since three patients did not have a substance abuse problem it was easier for the therapists and these three patients to generate peer pressure on those who did. If all the patients had believed their substance abuse was not a problem, the therapist would not have had any support. Social psychology research indicates minority opinions tend to change toward those of the majority. With court-committed patients who may not realize their need for treatment it therefore may be more productive, in certain situations, if the deviate opinion is in the minority than in the majority. In contrast, groups that have the same problem and admit their need for treatment frequently have greater group cohesiveness such as Alcoholics Anonymous. A major advantage of a music therapy intervention such as the rock band with court-committed patients is its ability to elicit and reinforce appropriate behavior even if the patients do not realize their need for treatment.

Patients with diversified problems. Occasionally the necessities of reality may dictate that music therapists do group therapy with patients having diversified or even disparate problems. We have found multimodal music therapy to be quiet flexible in such situations. Following is an example of a Group BASIC I.D. designed for Dick, Ben, and Victor, three adult psychiatric patients attending weekly music therapy sessions at the university music therapy clinic who were required to have group therapy by the referring agency.

GROUP BASIC I.D.

MODALITY	PROBLEMS	
Behavior	B-1:	Lack of – Dick – or inappropriate assertiveness – Victor
Affect	A-1:	Has difficulty with either expressing or identifying emotions – Dick
	A-3:	Low frustration tolerance that may result in verbal or physical aggression when frustrated – Victor
Sensation	NA	
Imagery	NA	
Cognitive	C-3:	Lacks problem solving skills – Dick
	C-9:	Gives up easily when solving problems; easily frustrated – Victor
	C-2:	Does not trust peers; does not like or trust others – Victor
Interpersonal	IS-6:	Difficulty talking with or sharing personal information with the group – Ben
	IS-7:	Has difficulty being accepted in groups or by community – Dick
	IS-1:	Isolative and feels very uneasy in group discussion – Ben
	IS-4:	Lacks leisure skills – Dick
	IS-9:	Inappropriate relationships with the opposite sex (doesn't say the right things) – Ben, Victor
Drugs	D-2.1:	Does not exercise regularly – Dick
	D-2.3:	Insomnia – Dick
	D-2.4:	Lack of muscular endurance (lower extremities) – Ben

A review of the PMTQs indicated Dick, Ben, and Victor had different problems that would need to be addressed during group therapy. However, the music assessment also indicated they all had positive attitudes toward participation in group music activities.

Because of the ability of many group music activities to simultaneously address different patient problems and modalities, the patients had a productive group therapy experience. The above Group BASIC I.D. was presented to the patients following its construction, and music therapy interventions were subsequently designed for the problems the patients indicated a desire to work on. One intervention used was the Multichord nontraditional guitar group (Cassity, 1977). During rehearsals, Ben gained experience at increasing his assertiveness, and Victor's assertiveness became more appropriate as they discussed the song lyrics and critiqued the group performances (Behavior); Ben shared personal information with the group and experienced group acceptance to counteract his withdrawal and feelings of uneasiness in group discussion (Interpersonal); Victor was given experience at pinpointing and offering appropriate solutions to problems of characters described in song lyrics to treat his low frustration tolerance and past failure at solving problems involving other people (Cognitive); Dick, because of his inability to identify and express feelings was given experience at identifying feelings projected in the songs, and at expressing the appropriate feeling when playing the song on the guitar (Affect); Scott's successful experience at playing the guitar helped counteract his depression (Affect) and provided a healthy coping mechanism (valued leisure skill).

Other group music therapy situations. It should be emphasized that the multimodal music therapy procedures presented in this manual, including the above group therapy procedures, are not meant to be rigidly adhered to. Multimodal music therapy should be considered a resource music therapist can *adapt* to their needs. The above information about group music therapy therefore may need to be adapted to meet the needs of the individual music therapist. It may be unnecessary to administer the PMTQ if the therapist feels sufficient assessment information already exists to write program plans for patients. Very large patient groups would likely present a need to design a more abbreviated evaluation format. The authors have used answer sheets to record individual patient responses when administering the PMTQ to large numbers of patients. Answer sheets have been placed behind each PMTQ in the Appendixes of this book. With patients who are high functioning enough, the therapist may need to administer the PMTQ in a group by letting each patient complete his own PMTQ. The major strength of multimodal music therapy however, is that it provides a systematic format for therapists who are having trouble obtaining adequate assessments, or with formulating individualized goals and objectives for group music therapy.

CHAPTER 11

BRIEF THERAPY
Short-Term Music Therapy

Because of changes in health care such as cost containment, managed health care, and health maintenance organizations (HMOs), music therapists are encountering an increasing number of settings in which it is necessary to have short-term treatment goals and objectives. According to Lazarus and Fay (1990), "One may predict that the 1990s will be an era in which brief therapies will proliferate and therapist accountability will be accentuated" (p. 41). Although music therapists may be asked to provide active treatment in as little as one session, in other settings brief therapy ranges upward to 40–50 sessions with a median duration of 20 sessions (Lazarus & Fay, 1990). Twenty sessions may be the most practical number of sessions in terms of reimbursement since "...many HMOs and insurance plans provide for brief treatment of up to 20 sessions" (Lazarus & Fay, 1990, p. 42). Multimodal therapy by its very nature is short-term therapy since 20 sessions is the average length of treatment. According to Lazarus and Fay (1990) the number of sessions in multimodal therapy could be reduced to as few as 10.

Although some may discount the effectiveness of short-term treatment, studies suggest that for many patients, short-term treatment has been effective in terms of achieving goals such as other and self awareness, clear thinking, socialization, personal effectiveness, self-esteem, and hopefulness (Hoge & McLoughlin, 1991; Liberman & Strauss, 1986). It is important to learn techniques of short-term treatment however, because long-term goals and objectives in a short-term setting is a prescription for therapist-patient frustration and failure.

The ability to plan a short-term treatment program is heavily dependent upon a knowledge of how the program will be evaluated. Treatment programs are evaluated in terms of whether the care is *appropriate* (clinically necessary) for the condition, the provider is *competent* to provide that care, the care is *cost-efficient,* the care is *accessible,* the care is *safe,* and the *patient is satisfied* (Goodman, Brown, & Deitz, 1992). For most music therapists therefore, the task is to design music therapy interventions that are appropriate, cost-efficient, and that result in patient satisfaction.

The first step in designing appropriate interventions is to conduct an initial assessment of the patient. Assessment information may include the patient's diagnosis, symptoms, and a description of the problems that led to the patient's admission to the facility. Why is the patient seeking treatment at this time? Where is the patient "stuck" and what would it take to get the patient "unstuck"? Whether or not to administer the PMTQ would depend upon the amount of time available, or whether there is sufficient information for music therapy program planning. However, the BASIC I.D. does provide a good brief format for organizing the patient's problems. Priority should be given to listing problems that can be treated with short-term goals and objectives since the overall focus is to stabilize the patient as soon as possible. Good treatment planning focuses on specific symptoms or problems (behaviorally defined and measurable) that support a medical necessity. Problems involving treatment planning are most frequently attributed to inadequate assessment, general or vague plans that are often unrelated to the patient's problems, plans that are not individualized, overly ambitious plans that cannot be achieved in the time frame allotted, plans that target further problems that are unnecessary for the patient's immediate treatment, failure to inform the patient of the treatment plan, and lack of compliance of the treatment plan with the institutional program or protocols (Sterman, 1993).

Therapeutic Factors Promoting Change in Short-Term Settings

Hoge and McLoughlin (1991) summarized the results of five studies reporting patient perceptions of therapeutic factors important for group therapy in short-term settings. The patients, described as low-functioning, including the "...most seriously and acutely ill" (Hoge & McLoughlin, 1991, p. 154), appeared to approximate the level of patient most music therapists treat (Cassity & Cassity, 1994). Seven factors the patients reported as most important at promoting therapeutic change were *self-responsibility, self-understanding, instillation of hope, group cohesiveness, catharsis, altruism*, and *universality*. Group therapy enabled the patients to discharge the overwhelming negative affect frequently experienced at the time of admission, or talk about negative experiences (catharsis), to realize that others have similar problems that may even be worse than their own problems (universality), and to offer mutual support to other group members at a time when they believe they had nothing to offer others (altruism). Self-understanding results when patients are able to perceive their problems more clearly and cope with them. In the process of discovering that others also have problems the patient's perspective often changes from *I am a terrible person* to *I have terrible problems*. The patient begins to understand that it is human to have problems. Group cohesiveness can be cultivated in acute treatment settings because patients have numerous hours throughout the day to participate in group activities resulting in increased verbal interaction that can continue beyond the ward (Hoge and McLoughlin, 1991; Maxmen, 1984). The instillation of hope usually is a derivative of the other therapeutic factors. Patients commonly arrive for treatment demoralized and hopeless. As they discharge negative affect, accept greater self-responsibility, and experience greater self-understanding, altruism, and universality patients become more confident and successful at coping with their problems both in the treatment setting and especially in the community. Contrary to traditional psychotherapeutic thought, therapists in short-term settings must acknowledge that most patient change will occur in the community after discharge.

Therapeutic Techniques for Short-Term Settings

To maximize the above therapeutic factors, Hoge and McLoughlin (1991) recommend the following techniques for group therapy in short-term treatment settings. At the beginning of each session behaviorally defined expectations should be stated for the group. Patients may be expected to discuss problems that led to their admission, or in the case of a lower functioning patient, make one relevant statement during the discussion. Once the session begins the therapist may use a variety of group intervention strategies such as encouraging patients to talk about their problems, setting limits to help patients control their behavioral excesses while encouraging the participation of quiet members, directing the group discussion toward problem solving, and encouraging appropriate expression of affect. As the discussion unfolds the therapist prompts responses in the form of questions and personal reactions to statements, and gives advice and support. The therapist can promote universality by underscoring the similarity of patient problems, and promote altruism by acknowledging the contributions the members are making to one another. Group cohesiveness can be promoted by therapist acceptance of all the group members, and patient hope can be instilled by the therapist indirectly and overtly projecting the attitude that each patient will recover from their crisis and learn to manage their problems. "The objective of the group is to facilitate crisis resolution, not personality change." (Hoge & McLoughlin, 1991, p. 156).

Music Therapy in Short-Term Settings

An inspection of the patient problems and music therapy interventions in this manual will reveal many patient problems and music therapy interventions suitable for short-term treatment. The above techniques for short-term settings may be readily adapted to group music therapy activities, especially lyric discussion activities focused on patient problems. Nontraditional instrumental ensembles designed for instant success are excellent for cultivating group cohesiveness, and increasing verbal interaction and self-responsibility among patients. Cassity (1994), using Unichord nontraditional guitar technique, significantly increased the group cohesiveness of adult psychiatric patients in as few as 10 sessions. The number of sessions required to increase group cohesiveness may be reduced even more by using simpler nontraditional techniques such as the EZ Chord or the Multichord guitar technique (Cassity, 1977), and color-coded techniques for playing the keyboard. The increased cohesiveness and verbalization generated by a performance group often generalizes to other treatment groups, such as music therapy groups that are more discussion oriented (such as lyric discussion) and to psychotherapy groups conducted by other professionals.

Another major role of music therapy in the short-term treatment setting is its role in preventative treatment (Shultis, O'Brien, DeBlasio, & Jasko, 1994). Preventing future hospitalization is a major cost containment incentive for managed health care. The music therapist can provide the patient with numerous techniques they can use in the community as assistive devices for coping with their problems. Such techniques are consistent with the above model that encourages patients to assume responsibility for their own health (self-responsibility). Examples of such techniques are educating the patient about how to use music in stress and pain management (Shultis et al., 1994) and in developing healthy methods of coping (e.g., healthy leisure skills). For patients having difficulty coping with stress, tension, anxiety, or pain the music therapist can provide instruction in muscle relaxation techniques to music, provide information about types of music conducive to relaxation, and instruct the patient in guided imagery techniques as self-help exercises for controlling pain (Wylie & Blom, 1986). Patients also need to be made aware of the mind/body connection in relation to the impact of the emotions on mental and physical health (Shultis et al., 1994). For example, a patient's music preference often reflects his or her diagnosis, and may even perpetuate it. Depressed clients choose melancholic songs, substance-abuse clients choose songs that remind them of previous *highs*, and children and adolescents with a history of sexual abuse, violence, and drug abuse often choose music concerned with Satanism, violence, sex, and drugs (Metzger, 1986). The lyrics of such music often reinforce rather than discourage inappropriate behavior, and therefore may be antagonistic to healthy post-hospital adjustment. Possible short-term treatment goals and objectives therefore could be focused toward assisting patients with recognizing songs that contribute to their problems, and in selecting songs within their preferred style of music, that represent healthy solutions to their problems.

Following is an example of a Multimodal Music Therapy Profile for Ron, a male adolescent, age 13 receiving short-term treatment. Since the music therapist did not have access to Ron's treatment records and therefore lacked sufficient information for program planning, the PMTQ for adolescents was administered to obtain immediate assessment information.

Multimodal Music Therapy Profile: *Ron*

I. MUSIC PREFERENCES

Ron strongly prefers popular and rock music. He indicated a strong dislike for country, folk, and religious music. He was neutral about jazz. Ron's *favorite groups* were AC-DC and Aero Smith. Ron expressed a desire to learn to play the drums and to perform for others. He also indicated a desire to learn to write music.

II. MULTIMODAL PROBLEM ANALYSIS

Affect	Problem	Music Therapy Intervention
A-2	Exhibits anger and rage	• Have patient select a song expressing the anger being felt. Follow by having the patient identify personal, appropriate alternatives for ventilating the anger.
A-3; A-4	Experiences stress reactions and excessive anxiety.	• Teach progressive muscle relaxation with or without background music. • Teach self-help guided imagery (GIM) to visualize successful involvement in stressful situations. Assist patient in identifying relaxing music; discuss appropriate stress resolution techniques. • Teach self-help GIM to imagine anxious situations then a positive outcome; discuss. • Instruct in use of biofeedback monitor and background music to reduce anxiety.
A-5	Poor impulse control	• Reduce negative comments from peers by improving peer or interpersonal relationships – assign patient to play trap drum set in patient rock band. Suggested song: *Lean on Me*. • Arrange for possible drum lessons in the community upon release from facility to increase frustration tolerance (if possible, refer to local music therapist).

Interpersonal	Problem	Music Therapy Intervention
IS-2	Lacks awareness of others	• Encourage more appropriate peer interactions during above lyric discussion group and in above rock band. • Conduct lyric discussions about songs which identify (1) destructive defenses and (2) positive self-protection in relationships.
IS-4	Lacks healthy methods of coping (poor leisure skills); spends time with gangs.	• Investigate the possibility of the patient playing drums in the school band.

Cognitive	Problem	Music Therapy Intervention
C-1	Low self-confidence; usually fails	• Insure success in above rock band; emphasize importance of success in community drum lessons and school band.
C-2; C-3	Lacks problem solving skills and gives up easily (low frustration tolerance).	• Ask the patient to imagine problem-solving situations and to mentally rehearse being in control as part of the above GIM self-help instruction. • Relate successful problem-solving behavior in rock band or during drum lessons to other life situations to promote generalization.
C-5	Does not respond well to constructive criticism.	• Have the rock band members take turns constructively critiquing the performance. • Recommend that acceptance of constructive criticism be noted during community drum lessons or in school band.
C-8; C-9; C-10	Ongoing conflict with parents.	• Discuss ways to solve family problems in above lyric discussion intervention; follow with letter-writing intervention described in manual. • Implement improvisational interventions in manual if time permits.

Drugs	Problem	Music Therapy Intervention
D-1.1	Believes drugs won't hurt him.	• Lyric analysis of songs portraying the negative effects of drugs (e.g., *A New Drug*, Huey Lewis and The News). • If time permits, role play consequences and negative behaviors associated with drug usage to increase self-awareness.

Behavior	Problem	Music Therapy Intervention
	NA	No problems indicated

III. POST INTERVIEW OBSERVATIONS – NA

Numerous music therapy interventions involving Ron could be accomplished in a single session. Such interventions include arranging for possible community drum lessons or possible inclusion in the public school music program, and prescribing the home use of self-instructional GIM, relaxing music, or progressive muscle relaxation with music recordings. Letting a patient play a preferred music instrument for a single session may lead to a desire to take lessons upon leaving the facility. Lyric discussion interventions also can be conducted in a single session.

Post Interview Observations were not administered to Ron because the PMTQ was administered to a group of patients of whom Ron was a member, and each patient completed their own PMTQ as the therapist supervised. The reason for this procedure was that there was not enough time to administer the PMTQ to each client on a one-to-one basis because of the shortage of session time. It has been our experience that if patients are high functioning enough, they are able to complete the PMTQ in a group situation. The above Multimodal Music Therapy Profile provides ample information for the implementation of a short-term music therapy program.

Ron was seen for seven sessions. In brief multimodal therapy, the clinician does not attempt to remediate every problem on the BASIC I.D., but with the client, selects three to five primary problems to target. As a result of working on primary problems, a ripple effect frequently will be observed in which the patient may also improve in the more secondary problems that are not directly targeted (Lazarus & Fay, 1990). As indicated previously, in a music therapy performance group such as the rock band, a somewhat greater number of problems may be targeted because of the interactive nature of the activity. Ron's music therapy program was designed to treat his primary problems of low frustration tolerance, anger, anxiety, stress reactions, poor impulse control, lack of awareness of others, unhealthy methods of coping, and unrealistic perceptions concerning drugs. The first half of the music therapy session focused on lyric discussion techniques to develop awareness of the negative effects of substance abuse, and the development of appropriate anger and stress resolution techniques. Homework assignments in the form of relaxation and GIM exercises also were given for managing anxiety and stress. Efforts also were made to involve Ron in community drum lessons or in a school or community band to promote more healthy methods of coping. During the second half of the session the rock band was employed to treat low frustration tolerance, inappropriate stress reactions, poor impulse control, and lack of awareness of others.

Ron's plan met the evaluation criteria of short-term treatment programming in that it was appropriate (clinically necessary) for his condition, it was cost-efficient, and he was satisfied with the treatment. The rock band was a great reinforcer as he looked forward to coming to music therapy each week. The plan also provided the therapist with a mechanism for fostering the therapeutic factors promoting change in short-term settings discussed above, by providing for the development of self-responsibility, self-understanding, instillation of hope, group cohesiveness, catharsis, altruism, and universality. Finally, Ron's plan recognized that the critical change in his behavior will occur in the community and therefore provided community supports to prevent further hospitalization.

The following reference list is provided for those who desire further information regarding short-term treatment.

References for Brief Therapy and Short-Term Psychotherapy

Adams, J. F., Piercy, F. P., & Jurich, J. A. (1991). Effects of solution focused therapy's "formula first session task" on compliance and outcome in family therapy. *Journal of Marital and Family Therapy, 17,* 277–290.

Appelbaum, S. A. (1975). Parkinson's law in psychotherapy. *International Journal of Psychoanalytic Psychotherapy, 4,* 426–436.

Baekeland, F., & Lundwall, L. (1975). Dropping out of treatment: A critical review. *Psychological Bulletin, 82,* 738–783.

Barber, J. (1990). Miracle cures? Therapeutic consequences of clinical demonstrations. In J. K. Zeig & S. G. Gilligan (Eds.), *Brief therapy: Myths, methods and metaphors* (pp. 437–442). New York: Brunner/ Mazel.

Barten, H. H. (1965). The 15-minute hour: A brief therapy in a military setting. *American Journal of Psychiatry, 122,* 565–567.

Bauer, G. P., & Kobos, J. C. (1993). *Brief therapy: Short term psychodynamic intervention.* Northvale, NJ: Aronson, Inc.

Berenbaum, H. (1969). Massed time-limit psychotherapy. *Psychotherapy: Theory, Research & Practice, 6,* 54–56.

Bloom, B. L. (1981). Focused single-session therapy: Initial development and evaluation. In S. H. Budman (Ed.), *Forms of brief therapy* (pp. 167–218). New York: Guilford Press.

Budman, S. H. (Ed.). (1981). Forms of brief therapy. New York: The Guilford Press.

Budman, S. H., & Gurman, A. S. (1988). *Theory and practice of brief therapy.* New York: The Guilford Press.

Budman, S. H., Hoyt, M. F., & Friedman, S. (Eds.). (1992). *The first session in brief therapy.* New York: Guilford Publications, Inc.

Burke, J. D., et al. (1979). Which short-term therapy? *Archives of General Psychiatry, 36,* 177–186.

Butcher, J. N., & Koss, M. P. (1978). Research on brief and crisis-oriented psychotherapies. In S. L. Garfield & A. E. Bergin (Eds.), *Handbook of psychotherapy and behavior change: An empirical analysis* (2nd Ed., pp. 725–768). New York: Wiley.

Cummings, N. A. (1977). Prolonged (ideal) versus short-term (realistic) psychotherapy. *Professional Psychology, 4,* 491–501.

Cummings, N. A., & Follette, W. T. (1968). Psychiatric services and medical utilization in a prepaid health plan setting: Part II. *Medical Care, 6,* 31–41.

Davanloo, H. (Ed.). (1978). *Basic principles and techniques in short-term dynamic psychotherapy.* New York: S. P. Medical & Scientific Books.

de Shazer, S. (1985). *Keys to solutions in brief therapy.* New York: Norton.

de Shazer, S. (1988). *Clues: Investigating solutions in brief therapy.* New York: Norton.

Dreiblatt, I. S., & Weatherly, D. (1965). An evaluation of the efficacy of brief contact therapy with hospitalized psychiatric patients. *Journal of Consulting Psychology, 29,* 513–519.

Edelstien, M. G. (1990). *Symptom analysis: A method of brief therapy.* New York: Norton.

Emery, G., & Campbell, J. (1986). *Rapid relief from emotional distress.* New York: Rawson Associates.

Frances, A., & Clarking, J. F. (1981). No treatment as the prescription of choice. *Archives of General Psychiatry, 38,* 542–545.

Frances, A., Clarking, J., & Perry, S. (1984). *Differential therapeutics in psychiatry: The art and science of treatment selection.* New York: Brunner/Mazel.

Goulding, M. M., & Goulding, R. L. (1979). *Changing lives through redecision therapy.* New York: Brunner/ Mazel (paperback: New York: Grove Press).

Gustafson, J. P. (1986). *The complex secret of brief psychotherapy.* New York: Norton.

Haley, J. (1973). *Problem-solving therapy.* San Francisco: Jossey-Bass.

Haley, J. (1973). *Uncommon therapy: The psychiatric techniques of Milton Erickson, M. D.* New York: Norton.

Haas, L. J., & Cummings, N. A. (1991). Managed outpatient mental health plans: Clinical, ethical and practical guidelines for participation. *Professional Psychology: Research and Practice, 22*(1), 45–51.

Hoge, M. A., & McLoughin, K. A. (1991). Group psychotherapy in acute treatment settings: Theory and technique. *Hospital and Community Psychiatry, 42,* 153–157.

Horowitz, M. J. (1976). *Stress response syndromes.* New York: Aronson.

Horowitz, M. J., Marmar, C., Krupnick, J., Wilner, N., Kaltreider, N., & Wallerstein, R. (1984). *Personality styles and brief psychotherapy.* New York: Basic Books.

Hoyt, M. F. (1979). Aspects of termination in a brief time limited psychotherapy. *Psychiatry, 42,* 208–219.

Hoyt, M. F. (1985). Therapist resistances to short-term dynamic psychotherapy. *Journal of the American Academy of Psychoanalysis, 13,* 93–112.

Hoyt, M. F. (1989). On time in brief therapy. In R. A. Wells & Giannetti (Eds.), *Handbook of the brief psychotherapies* (pp. 115–143). New York: Plenum Press.

Hoyt, M. F. (Ed.). (1994). *Constructive therapies.* New York: Guilford Publications, Inc.

Hoyt, M. F. (1995). *Brief therapy and managed care: Readings for contemporary practice.* San Francisco, CA: The Jossey-Bass.

Karon, B. P. (1995). Provisions of psychotherapy under managed health care: A growing crisis and national nightmare. *Professional Psychology: Research and Practice, 26*(1), 5–9.

Kellner, R., Neidhardt, J., Krakow, B., & Pathak, D. (1992). Changes in chronic nightmares after one session of desensitization or rehearsal instruction. *American Journal of Psychiatry, 149,* 659–663.

Koss, M. P., & Butcher, J. N. (1986). Research on brief psychotherapy. In S. L. Garfield & A. E. Bergin (Eds.), *Handbook of psychotherapy and behavior change* (pp. 627–670). New York: Wiley.

Lankton, S. R., & Erickson, K. K. (Eds.) (1994). The essence of a single-session success. *Ericksonian Monographs, 9,* 1–164.

Lazarus, A. A., & Fay, A. Brief psychotherapy: Tautology or oxymoron? (1990). In J. K. Zeigh & S. G. Gilligan (Eds.), *Brief therapy: Myths, methods, and metaphors* (pp. 36–51). New York: Brunner/Mazel.

Leibenluft, E., Tasman, A., & Green, S. A. (Eds.). (1993). *Less time to do more. Psychotherapy on the short term inpatient unit.* Washington, D. C.: American Psychiatric Press.

Lieberman, P. B., & Strauss, J. S. (1986). Brief psychiatric hospitalization: What are its effects? *American Journal of Psychiatry, 143,* 1557–1562.

MacKenzie, K. R. (1990). *Introduction to time-limited group psychotherapy.* Washington, D. C.: American Psychiatric Press, Inc.

Mahrer, A. R. (1990). *How to do experiential psychotherapy.* Ottawa, Canada: University of Ottawa Press.

Malan, D. H. (1976). *The frontier of brief psychotherapy.* New York: Plenum Press.

Malan, D., Heath, E., Bacal, H., & Balfour, F. (1975). Psychodynamic changes in untreated neurotic patients. II. Apparently genuine improvements. *Archives of General Psychiatry, 32,* 110–126.

Mann, M. (1973). *Time-limited psychotherapy.* Cambridge, MA: Harvard University Press.

Mann, J., & Goldman, R. (1982). *A casebook in time-limited psychotherapy.* New York: McGraw-Hill.

Margulies, A., & Havens, L. L. (1981). The initial encounter: What to do first? *American Journal of Psychiatry, 138,* 421–428.

Mumford, E., Schlesinger, H. J., Glass, G. V., Patrick, C., & Cuerdon, T. (1984). A new look at evidence about reduced cost of medical utilization following mental health treatment. *American Journal of Psychiatry, 141,* 1145–1158.

O'Hanlon, W. H., & Weiner-Davis, M. (1988). *In search of solutions: A new direction in psychotherapy.* New York: Norton.

O'Hanlon, W. H., & Hexum, A. L. (1990). *An uncommon casebook: The complete clinical work of Milton H. Erickson, M. D.* New York: Norton.

Oldman, J. M., & Russakoff, L. M. (1987). *Dynamic therapy in brief hospitalization.* North Vale, N J: Aronson, Inc.

Rockwell, W. J. K., & Pinkerton, R. S. (1982). Single-session psychotherapy. *American Journal of Psychotherapy, 36,* 32–40.

Rosenbaum, R. L. (1993). Heavy ideals: Strategic single-session hypnotherapy. In R. A. Wells & V. J. Giannetti (Eds.), *Casebook of the brief psychotherapies.* New York: Plenum Press.

Rosenbaum, R., Hoyt, M. F., & Talmon, M. (1990). The challenge of single-session therapies: Creating pivotal moments. In R. A. Wells & V. J. Giannetti (Eds.), *Handbook of the brief psychotherapies.* New York: Plenum Press.

Sautter, F., Heaney, C., & O'Neil, P. (1991). A problem solving approach to group psychotherapy in the inpatient milieu. *Hospital and Community Psychiatry, 42*(8), 814–817.

Shapiro, F. (1995). *Eye movement desensitization and reprocessing: Basic principles, protocols, and procedures.* New York: Guilford.

Shultis, C., O'Brien, A., DeBlasio, L., & Jasko, K. (1994, November). *Managed care and the role of the music therapist in acute psychiatric care.* Paper presented at the annual conference of the National Association for Music Therapy, Orlando, FL.

Sifneos, P. (1979). *Short-term psychotherapy and emotional crisis.* Cambridge, MA: Harvard University Press.

Sifneos, P. E. (1987). *Short-term dynamic psychotherapy* (Rev. Ed.). New York: Plenum Press.

Spoerl, O. H. (1975). Single-session psychotherapy. *Diseases of the Nervous System, 36,* 283–285.

Stern, S. (1993). Managed care, brief therapy and therapeutic integrity. *Psychotherapy, 30*(1), 162–175.

Strupp, H. H., & Binder, J. (1984). *Psychotherapy in a new key: Time-limited dynamic psychotherapy.* New York: Basic Books.

Talmon, M. (1990). *Single session therapy: Maximizing the effect of the first (and often only) therapeutic encounter.* San Francisco: Jossey-Bass.

Talmon, M. (1993). *Single session solutions.* Reading, MA: Addison-Wesley.

Talmon, M., Rosenbaum, R., Hoyt, M. F., & Short, L. (1990). Single *session therapy.* (Professional training videotape). Kansas City, MO: Golden Triad Films, Inc. (telephone 800-869-9454).

Wayne, G. J., & Koegler, R. R. (Eds.). (1966). *Emergency psychiatry and brief therapy.* Boston: Little Brown.

Weiner-Davis, M., de Shazer, S., & Gingerich, W. J. (1987). Building on pretreatment change to construct the therapeutic solution: An exploratory study. *Journal of Marital and Family Therapy, 13,* 359–363.

Wells, R. A. (1982). *Planned short-term treatment.* New York: Macmillan.

Wells, R. A., & Giannetti, V. J. (Eds.). (1990). *Handbook of the brief psychotherapies.* New York: Plenum Press.

Wells, R. A., & Giannetti, V. J. (Eds.). (1992). *Casebook of the brief psychotherapies.* New York: Plenum Press.

Wilson, G. T. (1981). Behavior therapy as a short-term therapeutic approach. In S. H. Budman (Ed.), *Forms of brief therapy.* New York: Guilford Press.

Winokur, M., & Dasberg, H. (1983). Teaching and learning short-term dynamic psychotherapy. *Bulletin of the Menninger Clinic, 47,* 36–52.

Wolberg, L. R. (Eds.). (1980). *Handbook of short-term psychotherapy.* New York: Thieme Stratton.

Zeig, J. K., & Gilligan, S. C. (Eds.). (1990). *Brief therapy: Myths, methods, and metaphors.* New York: Brunner/Mazel.

APPENDIX I

A. PSYCHIATRIC MUSIC THERAPY QUESTIONNAIRE: ADULTS
B. OPTIONAL ANSWER SHEET

PATIENT IDENTIFICATION FORM: Adults

NAME: _____ SEX: _____ AGE: _____

DATE: _____

FORMAL/PRIMARY DIAGNOSIS:

AXIS I: _____

AXIS II: _____

AXIS III: _____

AXIS IV: _____

AXIS V: Current GAF: _____ Highest GAF past year: _____

TOTAL NUMBER AND LENGTH OF STAYS OF PRIOR HOSPITALIZATIONS:

HOSPITAL   LENGTH OF STAY

_____   _____

_____   _____

_____   _____

LENGTH OF HOSPITALIZATION AT PRESENT FACILITY: _____

_____

TYPES OF MEDICATION TAKEN   *AND* DOSAGE PRESCRIBED

_____   _____

_____   _____

_____   _____

_____   _____

PSYCHIATRIC MUSIC THERAPY QUESTIONNAIRE
ADULTS

INSTRUCTIONS: Parts I and II of the following questionnaire are to be administered by the **examiner, or therapist, interviewing the examinee, or patient.** Part III, Post Interview Observations, will be completed by the examiner following termination of the interview, or Part II.

EXAMINER: A major purpose of therapy is to assist you with problems that may be interfering with your ability to enjoy life to the fullest. The purpose of this questionnaire therefore, is to assist you in recognizing problems or "bad habits" you may have and wish to get rid of. Since these questions are personal, you may be assured of complete confidentiality. NO ONE WILL SEE YOUR ANSWERS OTHER THAN THE THERAPISTS. If you do not care to answer these questions simply tell me you do not care to answer these questions.

I. MUSIC (viii)

1. EXAMINER: For the following styles of music tell me the number that indicates the degree you like each type of music. (Examiner gives the attached scale, like the one below, to the examinee.)

	Strongly Dislike	Dislike	Neutral	Like	Strongly Like
COUNTRY	1	2	3	4	5
POPULAR	1	2	3	4	5
ROCK	1	2	3	4	5
JAZZ	1	2	3	4	5
FOLK	1	2	3	4	5
RELIGIOUS	1	2	3	4	5
OTHER: _____	1	2	3	4	5

2. EXAMINER: Who is your favorite performer or composer?
(INSTRUCTION: Examiner writes in name below)

_____

INSTRUCTIONS FOR EXAMINER: Give the examinee the scale, like the one below, attached to this questionnaire. The examinee may then refer to the scale as necessary when choosing a number.

EXAMINER: I am going to read some statements. After each statement tell me the number from this scale that describes the extent you agree with the statement.

	Strongly Disagree	Disagree	Neutral	Agree	Strongly Agree
	1	2	3	4	5

3. ____ I would like to participate in a group sing-a-long with a pianist or guitarist accompanying the group. (viii)

4. ____ I would like to sing on stage before an audience.

5. ____ I would like to learn to play a musical instrument.

II. MULTIMODAL PROBLEM ANALYSIS

INSTRUCTIONS FOR EXAMINER: Let the examinee continue to keep the scale, like the one below. The examinee may then refer to the scale as necessary when choosing a number.

EXAMINER: I am going to read some statements. After each statement tell me the number from this scale that describes the extent you agree with the statement.

	Strongly Disagree	Disagree	Neutral	Agree	Strongly Agree
	1	2	3	4	5

Interpersonal (v)

1. ____ I would rather be alone than be with people. (IS-1)

2. ____ I find it hard to make friends.

3. ____ I have no close friends.

4. ____ It is easy for me to talk to people.

5. ____ It is hard for me to talk when in a group of people.

6. ____ I have trouble listening to others when they talk to me.

7. ____ I do not have a hobby; I rarely do something just for fun. (IS-2, IS-4)

8. ____ I would rather be alone or do nothing than to do something for fun with other people.

9. ____ There is not much to do in my spare time other than to sleep or watch television.

10. ____ I often get into trouble for not following directions, rules or regulations, or for not doing what I am suppose to do (e.g., smoking, eating, or drinking where prohibited). (IS-3)

11. ____ Friendships or relationships with other people usually do not last more than one year. (IS-5)

12. ____ I fight a lot with either my spouse (husband or wife) or family.

13. _____ I would feel very uneasy telling a group of people my likes, dislikes, and personal experiences. (IS-6)

14. _____ I have no difficulty being accepted by community groups (e.g., church, service groups) and with being invited to their events (e.g., parties, "get togethers"). (IS-7)

15. _____ I would rather sit behind the group members or sit alone than to sit with the group. (IS-8)

16. _____ I say the right things when trying to make friends with the opposite sex. (IS-9)

17. _____ Listening to the problems of others is boring; I become impatient. (IS-10)

Affect (iv)

18. _____ People cannot tell when I am happy, sad, or excited. (A-1)

19. _____ I rarely feel happy, sad, excited, or smile.

20. _____ I can easily tell when other people are happy, sad, or excited.

21. _____ I never worry about anything. (A-2)

22. _____ I never get angry or mad at people.

23. _____ I frequently experience feelings of anger and stress (A-3)

24. _____ I often hurt the feelings of my friends.

25. _____ I often hit other people. (A-3, A-10)

26. _____ I often feel like I have a tremendous amount of energy (i.e., difficulty sleeping, constantly moving and talking). (A-4)

27. _____ I often feel like I have no energy and feel very sad. (A-5)

28. _____ I frequently feel depressed or "down in the dumps."

29. _____ I frequently feel like killing or hurting myself. (A-6)

30. _____ I often wish I were dead.

31. _____ I experience a lot of anxiety (A-7).

32. _____ I often experience excessive anxiety from one or more of the following: present or past problems with other people, worry about the future (e.g., upcoming events), my life situation.

33. _____ I often experience excessive anxiety that frequently results in one or more of the following: inability to relax, muscle stiffness, sleep disturbance, worry, verbally talking about my problems to myself or others.

34. _____ It is easy for me to lose self-control and exhibit too much laughing, crying, or anger. (A-8)

35. _____ I often become very, very scared along with one or more of the following: I get panicky, my heart beats fast, I experience shortness of breath. (A-9)

36. _____ Sometimes I get so mad I could kill people. (A-10)

37. _____ Sometimes I get so mad I hit people.

38. _____ I frequently get mad when others give me advice.

39. _____ People often tell me I have a bad temper.

Cognitive (iv)

40. _____ I do not like myself. (C-1)

41. _____ I frequently call myself names such as "stupid," "idiot," or "dumb."

42. _____ I usually fail when I try to do something.

43. _____ People like me.

44. _____ I do not trust people. (C-2)

45. _____ Other people frequently lie about me.

46. _____ My problems are overwhelming; they can't be solved. (C-3)

47. _____ I have no trouble solving problems involving other people.

48. _____ I have trouble forgetting familiar things I should remember, such as my address, my telephone number, and names of close friends or family. (C-4)

49. _____ I do not remember things as well as most people, such as names, what I did yesterday, or things in my past. (C-5)

50. _____ I don't have any problems. (C-7)

51. _____ I do not wish to make any changes in my life; I am happy the way things are. (C-6, C-7, C-8)

52. _____ When I have a problem I would rather leave it unsolved than to spend a lot of time trying to solve it. (C-9)

53. _____ I get mad if I spend too much time trying to solve a problem.

54. _____ I have difficulty following directions. (C-10)

55. _____ I do not like to follow directions given by other people.

Behavior (iii)

56. _____ It seems I always do what others want to do rather than what I would like to do. (B-1)

57. _____ During group discussion I find it hard to express my own views on a topic, especially when they differ from the views of other group members.

58. _____ I have difficulty concentrating on one thing for very long. (B-2)

59. _____ I never interrupt others during discussions. (B-3)

60. _____ I make people mad by saying or doing the wrong things.

61. _____ I find it difficult to look at the person to whom I am speaking. (B-4)

62. _____ People get mad at me when I tell them what I want. (B-5)

63. _____ I would rather others make decisions about major changes in my life. (B-6)

64. _____ When people do something I don't like I may not cooperate with them (e.g., put things off they want me to do; be stubborn; half-heartedly participate in activities with them; not do as good a job for them as I would otherwise). (B-6)

65. _____ I may yell at people and call them derogatory names (e.g., stupid, dumb) when they do something I don't like. (B-7)

66. ____ I frequently lose my temper and argue with people.

67. ____ I frequently lose my temper and hit people. (B-8)

Drugs (substance use or abuse, physical, and communication) (v)

68. ____ I frequently drink excessively at home or at a bar. (D-1.1)

69. ____ I take drugs during my leisure time.

70. ____ I do not have a substance abuse problem (D-1.2)

71. ____ I take drugs or drink alcohol to cope with my life stress and for relaxation. (D-1.3)

72. ____ I do not exercise regularly. (D-2.1)

73. ____ I bathe daily. (D-2.2)

74. ____ I frequently experience one or more of the following: insomnia, lack of muscular endurance, awkwardness. (D-2.3 through D-2.7)

75. ____ People have trouble understanding me when I speak. (D-3.1 through D-3.7)

Note for Examiner: Item numbers 4, 14, 16, 20, 43, 47, 59 and 73 should be scored by reversing the scale. These items are stated in the affirmative rather than in the negative. Item number 70 should be scored by reversing the scale if other assessments indicate the patient presently does not have a substance abuse problem.

PART III. POST INTERVIEW OBSERVATIONS

INSTRUCTIONS: Following termination of the above interview and dismissal of the examinee, the examiner should record the following post interview impressions using the scale below. Items requiring observation in music activities should be completed after observing the patient in music activities.

Strongly Inadequate	Inadequate	Mediocre	Adequate	Strongly Adequate
1	2	3	4	5

76. ____ Rate the examinee's eye contact.

77. ____ Rate the examinee's posture.

78. ____ Rate the examinee's grooming.

79. ____ Did the examinee appear motivated to engage in music therapy?

80. ____ Did the examinee exhibit appropriate facial expressions?

81. ____ Did the examinee engage in conversation, or what degree of conversational skill was observed?

82. ____ How was the examinee's concentration?

83. ____ How was the examinee's attention span?

84. _____ How was the examinee's retention (e.g., Did test questions have to be repeated?)?

85. _____ How well does the examinee use music (e.g., artistic, to reflect feelings or emotions, as an escape)?

86. _____ Rate the examinee's overall attitude toward music.

87. _____ Rate your initial impression of the quality of the examinee's overall interpersonal relationships.

88. _____ How does the examinee perceive or solve problems during music activities?

89. _____ Rate your initial impression of the examinee's overall level of self-concept.

90. _____ Rate the examinee's abstracting ability (e.g., Did the examinee have trouble understanding the above questions? Did the examiner have to give a lot of examples?).

EXAMINER'S COMMENTS:

	Strongly Dislike	Dislike	Neutral	Like	Strongly Like
COUNTRY	1	2	3	4	5
POPULAR	1	2	3	4	5
ROCK	1	2	3	4	5
JAZZ	1	2	3	4	5
FOLK	1	2	3	4	5
RELIGIOUS	1	2	3	4	5
OTHER: _____	1	2	3	4	5

Strongly Disagree	Disagree	Neutral	Agree	Strongly Agree
1	2	3	4	5

OPTIONAL ANSWER SHEET

PATIENT IDENTIFICATION FORM: Adults

NAME: _____ SEX: _____ AGE: _____

DATE: _____ _____

FORMAL/PRIMARY DIAGNOSIS:

AXIS I: _____

AXIS II: _____

AXIS III: _____

AXIS IV: _____

AXIS V: Current GAF: _____ Highest GAF past year: _____

TOTAL NUMBER AND LENGTH OF STAYS OF PRIOR HOSPITALIZATIONS:

HOSPITAL   LENGTH OF STAY

_____   _____

_____   _____

_____   _____

LENGTH OF HOSPITALIZATION AT PRESENT FACILITY: _____

_____

TYPES OF MEDICATION TAKEN   *AND* DOSAGE PRESCRIBED

_____   _____

_____   _____

_____   _____

_____   _____

DIRECTIONS: USE THIS ANSWER SHEET TO RECORD ANSWERS TO THE *PMTQ* ADULTS

I. MUSIC

1. MUSIC STYLES

COUNTRY _____

POPULAR _____

ROCK_____

JAZZ _____

FOLK _____

RELIGIOUS_____

OTHER: _____

2. _____

3. _____

4. _____

5. _____

II. MULTIMODAL PROBLEM ANALYSIS

Interpersonal

1. _____
2. _____
3. _____
4. _____
5. _____
6. _____
7. _____
8. _____
9. _____
10. _____
11. _____
12. _____
13. _____
14. _____
15. _____
16. _____
17. _____

Affect

18. _____
19. _____
20. _____
21. _____
22. _____

23. _____
24. _____
25. _____
26. _____
27. _____
28. _____
29. _____
30. _____
31. _____
32. _____
33. _____
34. _____
35. _____
36. _____
37. _____
38. _____
39. _____

Cognitive

40. _____
41. _____
42. _____
43. _____
44. _____
45. _____
46. _____
47. _____
48. _____
49. _____
50. _____
51. _____
52. _____
53. _____
54. _____
55. _____

Behavior

56. _____
57. _____
58. _____
59. _____
60. _____
61. _____
62. _____

63. _____
64. _____
65. _____
66. _____
67. _____

Drugs (substance use or abuse, physical, and communication)

68. _____
69. _____
70. _____
71. _____
72. _____
73. _____
74. _____
75. _____

III. POST INTERVIEW OBSERVATIONS

76. _____
77. _____
78. _____
79. _____
80. _____
81. _____
82. _____
83. _____
84. _____
85. _____
86. _____
87. _____
88. _____
89. _____
90. _____

EXAMINER'S COMMENTS:

Appendix II

A. PSYCHIATRIC MUSIC THERAPY QUESTIONNAIRE: ADOLESCENTS
B. OPTIONAL ANSWER SHEET

PATIENT IDENTIFICATION FORM: Adolescents

NAME: _____ SEX: _____ AGE: _____

DATE: _____

FORMAL/PRIMARY DIAGNOSIS:

AXIS I: _____

AXIS II: _____

AXIS III: _____

AXIS IV: _____

AXIS V: Current GAF: _____ Highest GAF past year: _____

TOTAL NUMBER AND LENGTH OF STAYS OF PRIOR HOSPITALIZATIONS:

HOSPITAL   LENGTH OF STAY

_____   _____

_____   _____

_____   _____

LENGTH OF HOSPITALIZATION AT PRESENT FACILITY: _____

_____

TYPES OF MEDICATION TAKEN   *AND* DOSAGE PRESCRIBED

_____   _____

_____   _____

_____   _____

_____   _____

PSYCHIATRIC MUSIC THERAPY QUESTIONNAIRE
ADOLESCENTS

INSTRUCTIONS: Parts I and II of the following questionnaire are to be administered by the **examiner, or therapist, interviewing the examinee, or patient.** Part III, Post Interview Observations, will be completed by the examiner following termination of the interview, or Part II.

EXAMINER: A major purpose of therapy is to assist you with problems that may be interfering with your ability to enjoy life to the fullest. The purpose of this questionnaire therefore, is to assist you in recognizing problems or "bad habits" you may have and wish to get rid of. Since these questions are personal, you may be assured of complete confidentiality. NO ONE WILL SEE YOUR ANSWERS OTHER THAN THE THERAPISTS. If you do not care to answer these questions simply tell me you do not care to answer these questions.

I. MUSIC (x)

1. EXAMINER: For the following styles of music tell me the number that indicates the degree you like each type of music. (Examiner shows the following scale to the examinee).

	Strongly Dislike	Dislike	Neutral	Like	Strongly Like
COUNTRY	1	2	3	4	5
POPULAR	1	2	3	4	5
ROCK	1	2	3	4	5
JAZZ	1	2	3	4	5
FOLK	1	2	3	4	5
RELIGIOUS	1	2	3	4	5
OTHER: _____	1	2	3	4	5

2. EXAMINER: Who is your favorite performer or composer?
(INSTRUCTION: Examiner writes in name below)

INSTRUCTIONS FOR EXAMINER: Give the examinee the scale, like the one below, attached to this questionnaire. The examinee may then refer to the scale as necessary when choosing a number.

EXAMINER: I am going to read some statements. After each statement tell me the number from this scale that describes the extent you agree with the statement.

	Strongly Disagree	Disagree	Neutral	Agree	Strongly Agree
	1	2	3	4	5

3. ____ I would like to learn to play a musical instrument. (x)

4. ____ I would like to play a musical instrument for others.

5. ____ I would probably enjoy playing a musical instrument if I knew how (improvisation).

6. ____ I would like to participate in a group sing-a-long with a pianist or guitarist accompanying the group.

7. ____ I would like to learn to write music.

II. MULTIMODAL PROBLEM ANALYSIS

INSTRUCTIONS FOR EXAMINER: Let the examinee continue to keep the scale, like the one below. The examinee may then refer to the scale as necessary when choosing a number.

EXAMINER: I am going to read some statements. After each statement tell me the number from this scale that describes the extent you agree with the statement.

	Strongly Disagree	Disagree	Neutral	Agree	Strongly Agree
	1	2	3	4	5

Affect (vi)

1. ____ Other people know when I am happy, sad, or excited. (A-1)

2. ____ I rarely feel happy, sad, or excited.

3. ____ I can easily tell when other people are happy, sad, or excited.

4. ____ I often hurt the feelings of my friends. (A-2)

5. ____ I often hit other people.

6. ____ I often get mad at others.

7. ____ I often get mad at myself.

8. ____ I often hurt or feel like hurting myself.

9. ____ I often feel like destroying things that others have.

10. ____ I don't fight with or yell at others.

11. ____ I often feel like I am under a lot of stress. (A-3)

12. ____ Because of stress, I often experience one or more of the following: trouble sleeping, stomach aches, anxiety, and/or doing things I later regret.

13. _____ I experience a lot of anxiety. (A-4)

14. _____ My excessive anxiety frequently results from one or more of the following: present or past problems with other people; worry about the future (e.g., upcoming events).

15. _____ I frequently do things I later am sorry for. (A-5)

16. _____ It is hard for me to tell other people about bad things that happen to me. (A-6)

17. _____ It is hard for me to tell other people about good things that happen to me.

18. _____ I frequently feel depressed or "down in the dumps." (A-7)

19. _____ I frequently feel like killing myself. (A-8)

20. _____ It is easy to say nice things to people. (A-9)

Interpersonal (vi)

21. _____ I rarely get into trouble for not following rules and regulations, or not doing what I am suppose to do. (IS-1)

22. _____ I have trouble following directions (e.g., Stay in your chair; Finish your work; Work quietly; Be nice to others).

23. _____ I like to take turns and to share my things with others.

24. _____ I frequently get into trouble on and off hospital/school grounds.

25. _____ I like to tell others when they make a mistake. (IS-2)

26. _____ I frequently call people names such as "stupid," "idiot," or "dumb."

27. _____ I would rather be alone than be with people. (IS-3)

28. _____ I find it hard to make friends.

29. _____ I have no close friends.

30. _____ It is hard for me to talk to people.

31. _____ It is hard for me to talk when in a group of people.

32. _____ I spend most of my leisure time with a gang or in a bar. (IS-4)

33. _____ I do not have a hobby; I rarely do something just for fun (IS-4 through IS-5)

34. _____ I would rather be alone or do nothing than to do something with other people. (IS-5 through IS-6)

35. _____ I have trouble listening to others when they talk to me. (IS-6)

Cognitive (vi)

36. _____ I do not like myself. (C-1)

37. _____ I frequently call myself names such as "stupid," "idiot," or "dumb."

38. _____ I usually fail when I try to do something.

39. _____ People do not like me.

40. ____ I have a lot of problems. (C-2)

41. ____ I have no trouble solving problems involving other people.

42. ____ When I have a problem I would rather leave it unsolved than to spend a lot of time trying to solve it. (C-3)

43. ____ I get mad if I spend too much time trying to solve a problem.

44. ____ I do not trust other people. (C-4)

45. ____ Other people frequently lie about me.

46. ____ It bothers me for someone to tell me how I could do something better. (C-5)

47. ____ I never have any problems. (C-6)

48. ____ I have trouble keeping track of things; I frequently lose things (e.g., bills, records, money). (C-7)

49. ____ I am always fighting with my parents. (C-8 through C-10)

50. ____ I have no trouble making decisions (e.g., What I would like to do each day, what to eat for dinner, where to go, what music to listen to, what clothes to wear). (C-13)

Drugs (substance use or abuse) (vii)

51. ____ Drugs will not hurt me psychologically or physically. (D-1.1)

52. ____ I take drugs regularly. (D-1.1 through D-1.2)

53. ____ I do not have a substance abuse problem. (D-1.2)

54. ____ I take drugs or drink alcohol to cope with my life stress, unpleasant situations, or to block unpleasant feelings. (D-1.2)

Behavior (vi)

55. ____ It seems I always do what others want to do rather than what I would like to do. (B-1)

56. ____ During group discussion I find it hard to express my own views on a topic, especially when they differ from the views of other group members.

57. ____ I have difficulty concentrating on, or doing one thing for very long. (B-2, B-5)

58. ____ I usually leave or keep to myself when in a group. (B-3)

Note for Examiner: Item numbers 1, 3, 10, 20, 21, 23, 41, and 50 should be scored by reversing the scale. These items are stated in the affirmative rather than in the negative. Item number 53 should be scored by reversing the scale if other assessments indicate the patient presently does not have a substance abuse problem.

PART III. POST INTERVIEW OBSERVATIONS

INSTRUCTIONS: Following termination of the above interview and dismissal of the examinee, the examiner should record the following post interview impressions using the scale below.

Strongly Inadequate	Inadequate	Mediocre	Adequate	Strongly Adequate
1	2	3	4	5

59. _____ Rate your initial impression of the quality of examinee's overall interpersonal relationships.

60. _____ How well does the examinee use music (e.g., artistic; to reflect feelings or emotions; as an escape)?

61. _____ How does the examinee perceive, perpetuate, or solve problems during music activities?

62. _____ How was the examinee's concentration?

63. _____ How was the examinee's attention span?

64. _____ How was the examinee's retention (e.g., Did test questions have to be repeated?)?

65. _____ Rate the examinee's eye contact.

66. _____ Rate the examinee's posture.

67. _____ Rate the examinee's grooming.

68. _____ Did the examinee appear motivated to engage in music therapy?

69. _____ Did the examinee exhibit appropriate facial expressions?

70. _____ Did the examinee engage in conversation, or what degree of conversational skill was observed?

71. _____ Rate your initial impression of the examinee's overall level of self-concept.

72. _____ Rate the examinee's musical creativity or ability.

73. _____ Rate the examinee's overall attitude toward music.

EXAMINER'S COMMENTS:

	Strongly Dislike	Dislike	Neutral	Like	Strongly Like
COUNTRY	1	2	3	4	5
POPULAR	1	2	3	4	5
ROCK	1	2	3	4	5
JAZZ	1	2	3	4	5
FOLK	1	2	3	4	5
RELIGIOUS	1	2	3	4	5
OTHER: _____	1	2	3	4	5

Strongly Disagree	Disagree	Neutral	Agree	Strongly Agree
1	2	3	4	5

OPTIONAL ANSWER SHEET

PATIENT IDENTIFICATION FORM: Adolescents

NAME: _____ SEX: _____ AGE: _____

DATE: _____

FORMAL/PRIMARY DIAGNOSIS:

AXIS I: _____

AXIS II: _____

AXIS III: _____

AXIS IV: _____

AXIS V: Current GAF: _____ Highest GAF past year: _____

TOTAL NUMBER AND LENGTH OF STAYS OF PRIOR HOSPITALIZATIONS:

HOSPITAL   LENGTH OF STAY

_____   _____

_____   _____

_____   _____

LENGTH OF HOSPITALIZATION AT PRESENT FACILITY: _____

_____

TYPES OF MEDICATION TAKEN   *AND* DOSAGE PRESCRIBED

_____   _____

_____   _____

_____   _____

_____   _____

DIRECTIONS: USE THIS ANSWER SHEET TO RECORD ANSWERS TO THE *PMTQ* ADOLESCENTS

I. MUSIC

1. MUSIC STYLES
   COUNTRY _____
   POPULAR _____
   ROCK _____
   JAZZ _____
   FOLK _____
   RELIGIOUS _____
   OTHER: _____
2. _____
3. _____
4. _____
5. _____
6. _____
7. _____

II. MULTIMODAL PROBLEM ANALYSIS

Affect

1. _____
2. _____
3. _____
4. _____
5. _____
6. _____
7. _____
8. _____
9. _____
10. _____
11. _____
12. _____
13. _____
14. _____
15. _____
16. _____
17. _____
18. _____
19. _____
20. _____

Interpersonal

21. _____
22. _____
23. _____
24. _____
25. _____
26. _____
27. _____
28. _____
29. _____
30. _____
31. _____
32. _____
33. _____
34. _____
35. _____

Cognitive

36. _____
37. _____
38. _____
39. _____
40. _____
41. _____
42. _____
43. _____
44. _____
45. _____
46. _____
47. _____
48. _____
49. _____
50. _____

Drugs (substance use or abuse)

51. _____
52. _____
53. _____
54. _____

Behavior

55. _____
56. _____
57. _____
58. _____

III. POST INTERVIEW OBSERVATIONS

59. _____
60. _____
61. _____
62. _____
63. _____
64. _____
65. _____
66. _____
67. _____
68. _____
69. _____
70. _____
71. _____
72. _____
73. _____

EXAMINER'S COMMENTS:

Appendix III

PATIENT IDENTIFICATION FORM: Children

NAME: _____ SEX: _____ AGE: _____

DATE: _____

FORMAL/PRIMARY DIAGNOSIS:

AXIS I: _____

AXIS II: _____

AXIS III: _____

AXIS IV: _____

AXIS V: Current GAF: _____ Highest GAF past year: _____

TOTAL NUMBER AND LENGTH OF STAYS OF PRIOR HOSPITALIZATIONS:

HOSPITAL   LENGTH OF STAY

_____   _____

_____   _____

_____   _____

LENGTH OF HOSPITALIZATION AT PRESENT FACILITY: _____

_____

TYPES OF MEDICATION TAKEN   *AND* DOSAGE PRESCRIBED

_____   _____

_____   _____

_____   _____

_____   _____

PSYCHIATRIC MUSIC THERAPY QUESTIONNAIRE
CHILDREN

INSTRUCTIONS FOR EXAMINER: Parts I and II of the following questionnaire are to be administered by the examiner, or therapist, **interviewing a second person (examinee) who is familiar with the child**. The examinee is to be dismissed after finishing Part II.

EXAMINER: A major purpose of therapy is to assist persons with problems that may be interfering with their ability to experience success in life. The purpose of this questionnaire therefore, is to assist you in recognizing your child's problems or inappropriate behavior that you would like to see changed. Since these questions are personal, you may be assured of complete confidentiality. NO ONE WILL SEE YOUR ANSWERS OTHER THAN THE THERAPISTS. If you do not care to answer these questions simply tell me you do not care to answer these questions.

I. MUSIC (xi)

1. INSTRUCTION: Examiner gives the attached music preference scale to the examinee.

EXAMINER: For the following styles of music tell me the number that indicates the degree [PATIENT'S NAME] likes each type of music.

	Strongly Dislike	Dislike	Neutral	Like	Strongly Like
COUNTRY	1	2	3	4	5
POPULAR	1	2	3	4	5
ROCK	1	2	3	4	5
CHILDREN'S	1	2	3	4	5
FOLK	1	2	3	4	5
RELIGIOUS	1	2	3	4	5
OTHER: _____	1	2	3	4	5

2. EXAMINER: Can you tell me [PATIENT'S NAME]'s favorite recording, performer, or composer? (INSTRUCTION: Examiner writes in name below)

_____

INSTRUCTIONS FOR EXAMINER: Give the examinee the scale, like the one below, attached to this questionnaire. The examinee may then refer to the scale as necessary when choosing a number.

EXAMINER: I am going to read some statements. After each statement tell me the number from this scale that describes the extent the statement describes [PATIENT'S NAME].

Strongly Disagree	Disagree	Neutral	Agree	Strongly Agree
1	2	3	4	5

3. _____ Is able to identify characteristics of music such as style, slow or fast, which instruments are playing, and whether an instrument is playing or a person is singing. (xi)

4. _____ Sings melody in tune. (xi)

5. _____ Would enjoy playing a musical instrument. (xi)

6. _____ Would enjoy making up own movements to music. (xi)

II. MULTIMODAL PROBLEM ANALYSIS

INSTRUCTIONS FOR EXAMINER: Let the examinee continue to keep the scale, like the one below. The examinee may then refer to the scale as necessary when choosing a number.

EXAMINER: I am going to read some statements. After each statement tell me the number from this scale that describes the extent the statement describes [PATIENT'S NAME].

Strongly Disagree	Disagree	Neutral	Agree	Strongly Agree
1	2	3	4	5

Interpersonal (vii)

1. _____ Rarely gets into trouble for not following rules and regulations, or not doing what he/she is suppose to do. (IS-1)

2. _____ Has trouble following directions (e.g., Stay in your chair; Finish your work; Work quietly; Be nice to others).

3. _____ Exhibits disruptive outbursts such as temper tantrums to attract attention.

4. _____ Is liked by peers.

5. _____ Frequently calls others names such as "stupid," "idiot," or "dumb."

6. _____ Does not talk, or talks very little with peers. (IS-2)

7. _____ Does not participate or avoids participating in group activities with peers.

8. _____ Is shy, timid, and not interested in peers.

9. _____ Argues with peers. (IS-3)

10. _____ Does not cooperate when working or playing with peers.

11. _____ Likes to take turns and to share things with others. (IS-4)

12. _____ Does not pay attention to others while participating in structured activities. (IS-5)

13. _____ Speaks too softly to be heard by others. (IS-6)

14. _____ Demonstrates good leadership skills (e.g., team captain). (IS-7)

15. _____ Does not express or respond to greetings or closings (e.g., good-byes, hellos). (IS-8)

Behavior (vii)

16. _____ Does not express needs or wants to others. (B-1)

17. _____ Goes along with the group instead of stating own opinions or feelings.

18. _____ Does not stay on task, is too easily distracted, and has poor concentration. (B-2)

19. _____ Grabs things from others instead of sharing or taking turns. (B-3)

20. _____ Hits peers. (B-4)

21. _____ Has poor eye contact; does not look at person speaking, or when speaking; looks away or down when speaking or being spoken to. (B-5)

Drugs (Motor) (viii)

22. _____ Awkward when attempting common movements such as walking. (D-1.1)

23. _____ Runs into people when in a group.

24. _____ Cannot use fingers to perform tasks as well as peers (e.g., picking up coins, grasping a pencil, dialing a telephone number, turning pages of a book [finger dexterity]). (D-1.2 through D-1.3)

25. _____ Catches ball, claps hands, hits toy drum with ease. (D-1.4)

26. _____ Often drops objects causing disruptions to others and embarrassment to self. (D-1.5)

27. _____ Cannot recall recent family events such as a trip to the park. (D-2.1)

28. _____ Has trouble imitating speech or sounds. (D-2.2)

29. _____ Talks too loud. (D-2.3)

30. _____ Does not pronounce words clearly. (D-2.4)

31 _____ Has trouble comprehending what is said to him or her. (D-2.5)

Cognitive (vii)

32. _____ Has trouble with following directions. (C-1)

33. _____ Understands concepts such as left and right, behind, in front of, and next to, or over, under, around, and through. (C-2)

34. _____ Makes negative comments about self, such as "I'm dumb" or "I'm not very smart." (C-3)

35. _____ Refuses to participate in group or individual activities because of a lack of self-confidence (e.g., afraid of failure or ridicule). (C-3)

36. _____ Exhibits one or more of the following when performing tasks: disorganized rather than goal directed; fast without concern for quality rather than slow and deliberate; gives up easily rather than demonstrating perseverance; inaccurate rather than accurate. (C-4)

37. _____ Makes derogatory comments to peers if they don't do what he or she wants. (C-5)

38. _____ Has trouble telling what time it is, or the day of the week. (C-6)

39. _____ Has trouble counting money. (C-7)

40. _____ Has trouble memorizing the letters of the alphabet. (C-8)

41. _____ Has trouble counting. (C-9)

Affect (vii)

42. _____ Other people know when he or she is happy, sad, or excited. (A-1)

43. _____ Shows little or no emotion (e.g., happy, sad, or excited).

44. _____ Can easily tell when other people are happy, sad, or excited.

45. _____ Has trouble describing how others feel.

46. _____ Exhibits too many emotional extremes (e.g., laughing or crying, happy or sad).

47. _____ Emotions which are exhibited are frequently inappropriate for the occasion or situation (e.g., laughs in sad situations or when sad, cries when happy or in happy situations).

Note for Examiner: The above item numbers 1, 4, 11, 14, 25, 33, 42, and 44 should be scored by reversing the scale. These items are stated in the affirmative rather than in the negative.

PART III. POST INTERVIEW OBSERVATIONS

INSTRUCTIONS FOR THE EXAMINER: Part III, Post Interview Observations, is to be completed by the music therapist after observing the patient in music therapy. Rate items 48 through 62 using the following scale.

Strongly Inadequate	Inadequate	Mediocre	Adequate	Strongly Adequate
1	2	3	4	5

48. _____ Concentration

49. _____ Attention span

50. _____ Retention

51. _____ Interpersonal relationships

52. _____ Eye contact

53. _____ Posture

54. _____ Grooming

55. _____ Motivation to engage in music therapy

56. _____ Appropriate facial expressions

57. _____ Engages in conversation; degree of conversational skill

58. _____ Perceives and solves problems during music activities

59. _____ Uses music appropriately (e.g., artistic, to reflect feelings or emotions, as an escape)

60. _____ Musical creativity or ability

61. _____ Overall attitude toward music

62. _____ Rhythmic ability

63. Does the patient have any handicapping conditions that may impair activity participation?

YES   NO   (CIRCLE ONE)

(If YES, explain below under COMMENTS)

EXAMINER'S COMMENTS:

	Strongly Dislike	Dislike	Neutral	Like	Strongly Like
COUNTRY	1	2	3	4	5
POPULAR	1	2	3	4	5
ROCK	1	2	3	4	5
CHILDREN'S	1	2	3	4	5
FOLK	1	2	3	4	5
RELIGIOUS	1	2	3	4	5
OTHER: _____	1	2	3	4	5

Strongly Disagree	Disagree	Neutral	Agree	Strongly Agree
1	2	3	4	5

OPTIONAL ANSWER SHEET

PATIENT IDENTIFICATION FORM: Children

NAME: _____ SEX: _____ AGE: _____

DATE: _____

FORMAL/PRIMARY DIAGNOSIS:

AXIS I: _____

AXIS II: _____

AXIS III: _____

AXIS IV: _____

AXIS V: Current GAF: _____   Highest GAF past year: _____

TOTAL NUMBER AND LENGTH OF STAYS OF PRIOR HOSPITALIZATIONS:

HOSPITAL   LENGTH OF STAY

_____   _____

_____   _____

_____   _____

LENGTH OF HOSPITALIZATION AT PRESENT FACILITY: _____

_____

TYPES OF MEDICATION TAKEN   *AND* DOSAGE PRESCRIBED

_____   _____

_____   _____

_____   _____

_____   _____

DIRECTIONS: USE THIS ANSWER SHEET TO RECORD ANSWERS TO THE *PMTQ* CHILDREN

I. MUSIC

1. MUSIC STYLES
   COUNTRY _____
   POPULAR _____
   ROCK _____
   CHILDREN'S _____
   FOLK _____
   RELIGIOUS _____
   OTHER: _____
2. _____
3. _____
4. _____
5. _____
6. _____

II. MULTIMODAL PROBLEM ANALYSIS

Interpersonal

1. _____
2. _____
3. _____
4. _____
5. _____
6. _____
7. _____
8. _____
9. _____
10. _____
11. _____
12. _____
13. _____
14. _____
15. _____

Behavior

16. _____
17. _____
18. _____
19. _____
20. _____
21. _____

Drugs (Motor)

22. _____
23. _____
24. _____
25. _____
26. _____
27. _____
28. _____
29. _____
30. _____
31. _____

Cognitive

32. _____
33. _____
34. _____
35. _____
36. _____
37. _____
38. _____
39. _____
40. _____
41. _____

Affect

42. _____
43. _____
44. _____
45. _____
46. _____
47. _____

III. POST INTERVIEW OBSERVATIONS

48. _____
49. _____
50. _____
51. _____
52. _____
53. _____
54. _____
55. _____
56. _____
57. _____
58. _____
59. _____
60. _____
61. _____
62. _____
63. _____

EXAMINER'S COMMENTS:

Appendix IV

CLINICAL FORMS
ALTERNATE RECORDING FORMS

BASIC I.D.

MODALITY   PROBLEMS

Behavior

_____

_____

_____

Affect

_____

_____

_____

Sensation

_____

_____

_____

Imagery

_____

_____

_____

Cognitive

_____

_____

_____

Interpersonal

_____

_____

_____

Drugs

_____

_____

_____

Multimodal Music Therapy Profile: _____
(Adults)

I. MUSIC PREFERENCES

_____

_____

_____

II. MULTIMODAL PROBLEM ANALYSIS

Interpersonal	Problem	Music Therapy Intervention
___	_____	_____
___	_____	_____
___	_____	_____
___	_____	_____

Affect	Problem	Music Therapy Intervention
___	_____	_____
___	_____	_____
___	_____	_____
___	_____	_____

Cognitive	Problem	Music Therapy Intervention
___	_____	_____
___	_____	_____
___	_____	_____
___	_____	_____

Behavior	Problem	Music Therapy Intervention
___	_____	_____
___	_____	_____
___	_____	_____
___	_____	_____

Drugs	Problem	Music Therapy Intervention
___	_____	_____
___	_____	_____
___	_____	_____
___	_____	_____

III. POST INTERVIEW OBSERVATIONS

_____

_____

Multimodal Music Therapy Profile: _____
(Adolescents)

I. MUSIC PREFERENCES

_____

_____

_____

II. MULTIMODAL PROBLEM ANALYSIS

Affect	Problem	Music Therapy Intervention
____	____	____
____	____	____
____	____	____
____	____	____

Interpersonal	Problem	Music Therapy Intervention
____	____	____
____	____	____
____	____	____

Cognitive	Problem	Music Therapy Intervention
____	____	____
____	____	____
____	____	____

Drugs	Problem	Music Therapy Intervention
____	____	____
____	____	____
____	____	____

Behavior	Problem	Music Therapy Intervention
____	____	____
____	____	____
____	____	____

III. POST INTERVIEW OBSERVATIONS

_____

_____

Multimodal Music Therapy Profile: _____
(Children)

I. MUSIC PREFERENCES

_____

_____

_____

II. MULTIMODAL PROBLEM ANALYSIS

Interpersonal	Problem	Music Therapy Intervention
_____	_____	_____
_____	_____	_____
_____	_____	_____
_____	_____	_____

Behavior	Problem	Music Therapy Intervention
_____	_____	_____
_____	_____	_____
_____	_____	_____
_____	_____	_____

Drugs	Problem	Music Therapy Intervention
_____	_____	_____
_____	_____	_____
_____	_____	_____
_____	_____	_____

Cognitive	Problem	Music Therapy Intervention
_____	_____	_____
_____	_____	_____
_____	_____	_____
_____	_____	_____

Affect	Problem	Music Therapy Intervention
_____	_____	_____
_____	_____	_____
_____	_____	_____
_____	_____	_____

III. POST INTERVIEW OBSERVATIONS

_____

_____

MUSIC THERAPY INTERVENTION PLAN

NAME: _____ CASE NO: _____

DATE OF ASSESSMENT: _____

Music Therapy Goals and Objectives

Goal #__: _____

Goal Statement: _____

_____

Objective #__.__ Objective Statement:_____

_____

_____

_____

Person Responsible: _____

Date Started: _____ Date Ended: _____

Reason Ended:_____

_____

Objective #__.__ Objective Statement:_____

_____

_____

_____

Person Responsible: _____

Date Started: _____ Date Ended: _____

Reason Ended:_____

_____

Objective #__.__ Objective Statement:_____

_____

_____

_____

Person Responsible: _____

Date Started: _____ Date Ended: _____

Reason Ended:_____

_____

IMPLEMENTATION STRATEGY

NAME: _____   CASE NO: _____

DATE OF ASSESSMENT: _____

Objective #__.__: _____

_____

_____

Materials Needed: _____

_____

Reinforcement Schedule: _____

THERAPIST BEHAVIOR   PATIENT BEHAVIOR

Music Therapy Progress Report Chart

Name of Agency: _____

Patient Name: _____ Therapist Name: _____

Specify goal and objective being worked on in the space provided. Place the appropriate evaluation code under the session date to indicate whether or not the objective was met, if the patient or therapist was absent, or if there was insufficient time to work on the objective. Write a progress report for each session.

Goal #__: _____
_____

Objective #__.__: _____
_____
_____

Date: /   /   /   /   /   /
Progress:

EVALUATION:
Record a "+" for completion of objective.
Record a "P" for progress toward meeting the objective.
Record a "–" for not meeting objective.
Record an "A" for patient or therapist being absent
Record an "0" for insufficient time during the session to work on the objective.

Session Progress Report/Comments

_____
_____
_____
_____
_____
_____
_____
_____
_____
_____

Name of Agency: _____

Patient Name: _____ Date: _____

Therapist Name: _____

INDIVIDUALIZED INTERVENTION PLAN

Long-Term Goal #1: _____

    Short-Term Objective #__.__ : _____

_____

_____

    Short-Term Objective #__.__ : _____

_____

_____

    Short-Term Objective #__.__ : _____

_____

_____

Long-Term Goal #2: _____

    Short-Term Objective #__.__ : _____

_____

_____

    Short-Term Objective #__.__ : _____

_____

_____

    Short-Term Objective #__.__ : _____

_____

_____

Long-Term Goal #3: _____

    Short-Term Objective #__.__ : _____

_____

_____

    Short-Term Objective #__.__ : _____

_____

_____

    Short-Term Objective #__.__ : _____

_____

_____

Plan: _____

_____

_____

_____

Patient or Parent/Guardian Response to Intervention Plan:

_____

_____

I am in agreement with this plan, and agree to attend sessions regularly to allow for optimal benefit. If I must cancel a session, I agree to give advanced notice if possible.

Signatures:

_____

Patient or Parent/Guardian

_____

Therapist

Name of Agency: _____

Patient Name: _____ Therapist Name: _____

SESSION PROGRESS NOTE

Date   **Length and Time**   **Session Summary**

_____
_____
_____
_____
_____
_____
_____
_____
_____
_____

Object   **Code**   **Comment**

__.__: ( ) _____
_____
_____

__.__: ( ) _____
_____
_____

__.__: ( ) _____
_____
_____

__.__: ( ) _____
_____
_____

__.__: ( ) _____
_____
_____

__.__: ( ) _____
_____
_____

__.__: ( ) _____
_____
_____

REFERENCES

Adleman, E. J. (1985). Multimodal therapy and music therapy: Assessing and treating the whole person. *Music Therapy, 5,* 12–21.

American Music Therapy Association. (1998). *Standards of clinical practice.* Silver Spring, MD: Author.

American Psychiatric Association. (1987). *Diagnostic and statistical manual of mental disorders-revised (DSM-III-R).* Washington, DC: Author.

American Psychiatric Association. (1994). *Diagnostic and statistical manual of mental disorders, fourth edition (DSM-IV).* Washington, D C: Author.

Anderson, T. K., Cancelli, A. A., & Kratochwill, T. R. (1984). Self-reported assessment practices of school psychologists: Implications for training and practice. *Journal of School Psychology, 22,* 17–29.

Bandler, R., & Grinder, J. (1975). *The structure of magic: A book about language and therapy* (Vol. 1). Palo Alto, CA: Science and Behavior Books.

Blodgett, G., & Davis, D. (1994, November). *Reliability of the Psychiatric Music Therapy Questionnaire for Adults: A pilot study.* Paper presented at the annual conference of the National Association for Music Therapy, Orlando, FL.

Britten, B. (1946). *The young person's guide to the orchestra.*

Carmines, E. G., & Zeller, R. (1979). *Reliability and validity assessment.* Sage University Paper series on Quantitative Applications in the Social Sciences, Beverly Hills, CA: Sage Publications, Inc.

Cassity, M. D. (1977). Nontraditional guitar techniques for EMR and TMR residents in music therapy activities. *Journal of Music Therapy, 14,* 39–42.

Cassity, M. D. (1985). Techniques, procedures and practices employed in the assessment of adaptive and music behaviors of trainable mentally retarded children. *Dissertation Abstracts International, 46,* 10A. (Ann Arbor: University Microfilms International No. 85-27959, 2955.)

Cassity, M. D. (1994). The influence of a music therapy activity upon peer acceptance, group cohesiveness and interpersonal relationships of adult psychiatric patients. In J. M. Standley & C. A. Prickett (Eds.), *Research in music therapy: A tradition of excellence, outstanding reprints from the Journal of Music Therapy 1964–1993* (pp. 189–200). Silver Spring, MD: National Association for Music Therapy.

Cassity, M. D. (1995). Clinical applications of music therapy in domestic violence. *Directions in Mental Health Counseling, 5* (11), 3–13.

Cassity, M. D., & Cassity, J. E. (1994). Psychiatric music therapy assessment and treatment in clinical training facilities. *Journal of Music Therapy, 31,* 2–30.

Cassity, M. D., & Theobald, K. A. (1990). Domestic violence: Assessments and treatments employed by music therapists. *Journal of Music Therapy, 27,* 179–194.

Egan, G. (1990). *The skilled helper: A systematic approach to effective helping.* Belmont, CA: Brooks/Cole Publishing Company.

Ficken, T. (1976). The use of songwriting in a psychiatric setting. *Journal of Music Therapy, 13,* 163–172.

Gaston, E. T. (1968). Man and music. In E. T. Gaston (Ed.), *Music in therapy* (p. 27). New York: The Macmillan Company.

George, W. E. (1980). Measurement and evaluation of musical behaviors. In D. A. Hodges (Eds.), *Handbook of music psychology* (p. 294). Lawrence, KS: National Association for Music Therapy.

Goodman, M., Brown, I., & Deitz, P. (1992). *Managing managed care: A mental health practitioner's survival guide.* Washington, DC: American Psychiatric Press.

Gresham, F. M. (1984). Behavioral interviews in school psychology: Issues in psychometric adequacy and research. *School Psychology Review, 13,* 17–25.

Gronlund, N. E. (1973). *Preparing criterion-referenced tests for classroom instruction.* New York: The Macmillan Company.

Groth-Marnat, G. (1990). *Handbook of psychological assessment.* New York: John Wiley & Sons.

Hoge, M. A., & McLoughlin, K. A. (1991). Group psychotherapy in acute treatment settings: theory and technique. *Hospital and Community Psychiatry, 42*(2), 153–158.

Jensen, K. L., & McKinney, C. H. (1990). Undergraduate music therapy education and training: Current status and proposals for the future. *Journal of Music Therapy, 27*, 158–178.

Lazarus, A. A. (1976). *Multimodal behavior therapy.* New York: Springer.

Lazarus, A. A. (1989). *The practice of multimodal therapy.* Baltimore: The Johns Hopkins University Press.

Lazarus, A. A., & Fay, A. (1990). Brief psychology: Tautology or oxymoron? In J. K. Zeigh & S. G. Gilligan (Eds.), *Brief therapy: Myths, methods, and metaphors* (36–51). New York: Brunner/Mazel.

Liberman, P. B., & Strauss, J. S. (1986). Brief psychiatric hospitalization: What are its effects? *American Journal of Psychiatry, 143*, 1557–1562.

Lloyd, N. (1968). *The golden encyclopedia of music.* New York: Golden Press.

Maxmen, J. S. (1978). An educative model for in-patient group psychotherapy. *International Journal of Group Psychotherapy, 28*, 321–338.

Metzger, L. K. (1986). The selection of music for therapeutic use with adolescents and young adults. *Music Therapy Perspectives, 3*, 20–24.

Murray, A. (1994, November). *Reliability of the Psychiatric Music Therapy Questionnaire with psychiatric patients: A pilot study.* Paper presented at the annual conference of the National Association for Music Therapy, Orlando, FL.

Panell, R. C. & Laabs, G. J. (1979). Construction of a criterion-referenced, diagnostic test for an individualized instruction program. *Journal of Applied Psychology, 3*, 255–261.

Plach, T. (1980). *The creative use of music in group therapy.* Springfield, IL: Charles C. Thomas, Publisher.

Popham, W. J. (1978). *Criterion-referenced measurement.* Englewood Cliffs, NJ: Prentice-Hall, Inc.

Popham, W. J., & Husek, T. R. (1969). Implication of criterion-referenced measures. *Journal of Educational Measurement, 6*, 1–9.

Rubin, B. (1973). Music therapy in an outreach station of the Milwaukee County Mental Health Center. *Journal of Music Therapy, 10*, 201–204.

Schoenfeldt, L. F., Schoenfeldt, B. B., Acker, S. R., & Perlson, M. R. (1976). Content validity revisited: The development of a content-oriented test of industrial reading. *Journal of Applied Psychology, 61*, 581–588.

Schulberg, C. H. (1981). *The music therapy sourcebook.* New York: Human Sciences Press.

Shultis, C., O'Brien, A., DeBlasio, L., & Jasko, K. (1994, November). *Managed care and the role of the music therapist in acute psychiatric care.* Paper presented at the annual conference of the National Association for Music Therapy, Orlando, FL.

Sterman, P. (1993, January). *Promoting the culture of quality.* Paper presented at the Group Health Association of America Conference, Lake Tahoe, NV.

Swezey, R. W. (1981). *Individual performance assessment: An approach to criterion-referenced test development.* Reston, VA: Reston Publishing Company, Inc.

Thaut, M. H. (1994). The influence of music therapy interventions on self-rated changes in relaxation, affect, and thought in psychiatric prisoner-patients. In J. M. Standley & C. A. Prickett (Eds.), *Research in music therapy: A tradition of excellence. Outstanding reprints from the Journal of Music Therapy 1964–1993* (pp. 224–236). Silver Spring, MD: National Association for Music Therapy, Inc.

Unkefer, R. F. (1990). *Music therapy in the treatment of adults with mental disorders.* New York: Schirmer Books.

Weiten, W., & Lloyd, M. A. (1994). *Psychology applied to modern life.* Pacific Grove, CA: Brooks/Cole Publishing Company.

Wolfe, D. E., Burns, S., Stoll, M., & Wichmann, K. (1975). *Analysis of music therapy group procedures.* Minneapolis, MN: Golden Valley Health Center.

Wylie, M. E., & Blom, R. C. (1986). Guided imagery and music with hospice patients. *Music therapy perspectives, 3*, 25–28.

of related interest

Analytical Music Therapy
Edited by Johannes Th. Eschen
ISBN 1 84310 058 4

Case Study Designs in Music Therapy
Edited by David Aldridge
ISBN 184310 140 8

Songwriting
Methods, Techniques and Clinical Applications for Music Therapy Clinicians, Educators and Students
Edited by Felicity Baker and Tony Wigram
Foreword by Even Ruud
ISBN 1 84310 356 7

Clinical Applications of Music Therapy in Psychiatry
Edited by Tony Wigram and Jos De Backer
Foreword by Jan Peuskens
ISBN 1 85302 733 2

Clinical Applications of Music Therapy in Developmental Disability, Paediatrics and Neurology
Edited by Tony Wigram and Jos De Backer
Foreword by Colwyn Trevarthen
ISBN 1 85302 734 0

Music, Music Therapy and Trauma
International Perspectives
Edited by Julie P. Sutton
ISBN 1 84310 027 4